T0073443

Syphilis

Andrew P. Zbar

Syphilis

A Short Biography

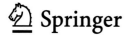 Springer

Andrew P. Zbar
University of Melbourne
Melbourne, VIC, Australia

ISBN 978-3-031-09773-7   ISBN 978-3-031-08968-8   (eBook)
https://doi.org/10.1007/978-3-031-08968-8

This Springer imprint is published by the registered company Springer Nature Switzerland AG
The registered company address is: Gewerbestrasse 11, 6330 Cham, Switzerland

To the spirit of Paul Ehrlich (1854–1915) who towered above others through his industry, the fertility of his mind and in how he conducted himself against prejudice.

Foreword

Andrew Zbar opens his treatise with a question: *Why write a book about syphilis?*
Initially, I thought this was merely rhetorical, to get the narrative rolling. But as the story of syphilis unfolds I realized this is a genuine enquiry, directed towards himself, and asked on behalf of the reader. The book itself becomes the answer.

And yet it is more than a book; the author has elevated the subject to be worthy of a 'biography', which, on the face of it, is a huge anthropomorphic leap for a bacterium, let alone a disease. Biographies are often written about great men and women, however, a quick scan of any reputable bookshop shelf will reveal that many, perhaps most, of the subjects of biographies are nowhere near as famous as syphilis. There are other biographies that hone in on the darker side of humanity and have as their subject true monsters—again syphilis is not out of place here.

This is a 'short' biography and cannot rival, in girth at least, those Winston Churchill door-stoppers that thump onto desks every couple of years. But it is a thorough and incisive exposé of a truly remarkable life-form that has influenced and even devastated the lives of any number of people who wind up the subject of a published biography. Syphilis may not be a person, but it is an intimate companion of humanity, in many ways unchanging, yet capricious enough to fight back when it seems not far from being silenced. While, personally, we would not choose the intimate company of the subject of this biography, we can enjoy vicariously many happy hours amongst these pages.

Zbar starts with the origins of the disease that has a long history of controversy. He deftly avoids getting bogged down with the 'who brought it back from where, and then gave it to whom' argument. Huge volumes of toner have been consumed arguing about the ancient European (or even older, African) origin of the disease as an alternative to the often-quoted arrival of syphilis from the Americas more than five centuries ago. Instead we first join the author on this journey in the company of the well-connected Girolamo Fracastoro. It was this Italian poet/physician who put the disease on the map, both metaphorically and literally, (achieving the latter by placing the blame at the feet of the French in the timeless xenophobic way we like naming diseases—the *morbus Gallicus*).

Next, we are invited to see the many guises of syphilis through a historical prism using magnificent descriptions from the past. The illustrations are carefully selected but it is the written record that brings the disease to life. Syphilis, as the descriptions attest, is truly versatile, 'malignant, occult and insidious'. With every scientific discovery of medical importance, there is often great hope and ambitious plans for disease eradication. Syphilis has had its share of pharmaceutical over-reachers, where a little knowledge quickly turns into arrogant bravado. And after hubris, failure often follows at great cost to reputations, but much more important to the poor patients who have followed these leaders down a road of quackery often out of desperation and blind hope. But in the middle of the last century, there arrived a great white powder to usher in the antibiotic era, and luckily for us penicillin remains the first choice of treatment for many serious illnesses including syphilis.

In the fifth chapter, we are shown the impact of syphilis on the arts both at a personal and cultural level. In the recording of stories about infectious diseases through the ages, the word 'romance' has often been hitched to tuberculosis, though given the mode of transmission one might think that syphilis is a better fit. In truth, I think we should leave the 'R' word well away from both of them. And yet syphilis has inspired a tremendous wealth of writing, from literature to satirical scorn, and portraiture, from epic canvasses to humorously vulgar cartoons making for a great and terrible record of a dreadful scourge.

Finally, there is, what will for many be the most important biographical details of the disease—the politics of syphilis. There is a powerful natural force that draws infectious diseases physicians, microbiologists and epidemiologists to calamitous infections especially if they cause large outbreaks of great morbidity. It can appear, to the unbiased observer, at least a bit uncaring, however, overwhelmingly the study of infectious diseases is undertaken with best intentions and by good people. But Tuskegee is now synonymous with one of the most heinous cases of medical malfeasance in history and now has a permanent place in medical ethics pedagogy, to remind us, emphatically, what not to do. It was a terrible irony that those whom the founders of that Institute set out to best serve, were the most beset victims of this wrongdoing. The story has been often told but in this chapter the misadventure is clearly laid bare under four apposite headings called the 'Medical', the 'Folkloric', the 'Factual' and the 'Racial Tuskegee'. Throughout the author takes a cool historian-scientist approach; but we can sense (and we share) his patent disgust.

So where does this book go in the library? History? Science? Medicine? It actually doesn't really matter, what's important is that the question that opened proceedings has been answered: *Why write a book about syphilis*? Because it is fascinating.

(…and by the way, it goes in the Biography section.)

Adam Jenney, M.B.B.S., Ph.D., F.R.A.C.P., F.R.C.P.A.
Head, Microbiology Unit
The Alfred Hospital
Monash University
Melbourne, Australia

Preface

Why write a book about Syphilis?

If we are to examine any infectious disease, the material aspects of its identification, its growth in culture, the clinical manifestations, its fastidious microbiological needs and habits and its treatment, are the domain of the scientist and the doctor. That too today along with the molecular information of its genetic backbone that has sequenced its unique genome. But the historical fingerprint of any disease like Syphilis can be found in its communicability, something more defining that lies outside the organism itself. Although it emerged in its most virulent form in the Renaissance, it is perhaps more impressionably aligned with the Victorian era (like another disease Tuberculosis) and it is through this association that it has become inculcated into the romantic literature and with its veil of secrecy, transcended social class.

This book is aimed at the presentation of more than the history of Syphilis as a distinct bacterium. I have entitled it a biography in order to render it more of an intimate account of its emergence and impact and to establish that connection between the organism itself and the social responses it provoked. Both most assuredly contribute to its definition. Chapter 1 examines the origins of European Syphilis, still somewhat shrouded in mystery and first lamented in the poetry of the Renaissance physician Girolamo Fracastoro (1478–1553). Chapter 2 considers the protean manifestations of disease and focuses on bizarre neuropsychiatric expressions of late Syphilis. Chapter 3 relates the history of the laboratory diagnosis of the disease and the quest for definitive anti-Syphilis therapy chronicling those who hitched their medical wagon to the curative properties of mercury, a drug-metal rooted in the era of alchemy and wizardry. Chapter 4 illustrates the impact of Syphilis on literature and in the arts, detailing the quirky notable history of some of its more renowned victims, both assured and presumptive. Chapter 5 deals with those whose prime interest in Syphilis was academic but whose ambitions clouded their goals leading them to behave in the most unethical manner in order to achieve their aims.

The Canadian physician Sir William Osler, (1849–1919) one of the founders of Johns Hopkins Hospital in Baltimore and one of the most highly cited of physicians had oft been quoted as saying *Know syphilis in all its manifestations and relations, and all other things clinical will be added unto you.* The statement is as true today as it ever was, just not as relevant in an age where the prevalence of disease is one where there is a diminishing law of returns.[1] Syphilis may not have killed as many people as the 'white plague' Tuberculosis but for the French medical historian Claude Quétel it has caused *the blackest ink to flow.*[2] As a disease, many of its representative specimens may now sit in museums calling to us with 500 years of collective memory but still it endures.

Melbourne, Australia   Andrew P. Zbar

---

[1] American, Canadian, English and Australasian medicine holds a soft spot for Osler particularly as he took up a post after Baltimore as the Regius Chair of Medicine at Oxford and then received a baronetcy. Osler through his aphorisms and pronouncements was, one might suggest preoccupied with his importance and his verbal legacy donating his personal library to McGill University in Montreal on the proviso that they dub it the *Bibliotheca Osleriana*. As a founding member of the American Anthropometric Society the last thing Osler did was to will his brain to the group (now held at the Wistar Institute Philadelphia) where it resides with the brains of the physicians William Pepper and Phillip Leidy, the palaeontologists Joseph Leidy and Edward Drinker Cope and (until the brain was dropped by a technician) the poet Walt Whitman.

[2] Claude Quétel. *The History of Syphilis.* Johns Hopkins University Press. 1990; p 2.

Acknowledgments

Just before the start of the COVID pandemic I was doing some research in Italy for a book about the history of anatomical illustration generated through human dissection. The trip ended with a visit to a museum in Florence *La Specola* that in three small room houses the exquisite wax models of complicated dissections that some believe are even more valuable in their ability to portray internal human anatomy than real-life dissections. The great ceroplastic masters like Clemente Susini (1754–1814) sculpted their simulacra from the intricate dissections of their anatomists, Felice Fontana (1730–1805) and Paolo Mascagni (1755–1815) using melted beeswax and the white Virgin insect wax that had been crushed from Japanese and Chinese scale insects shipped from as far away as Venice and Smyrna.

Some of the smallest but most extraordinary of these sculptures were made, however, a hundred years before by the ascetic Jesuit monk Gaetano Giulio Zumbo (1656–1701) where they can be found at the front of the exhibit. Here Zumbo created his remarkable pieces the *Theatres of Death* orchestrating tiny morbid figures in twisted agony to portray the realities of *La Peste* (the Plague) and *il morbo Gallicus* (the French disease so-called of Syphilis). In his diorama of *Syphilis*, there is the full panoply of a rampant medieval disease right down to one man his nose eaten away who laments the fate of others whose whole bodies have been devoured. This is a display of Biblical proportions. Devastating, penitent, God-fearing and historically retributive. It left a deep impression on me and I resolved to find out how this disfiguring disease arrived on to European shores and how it has mutated into something ignominious and even pedestrian. In my research, there are huge holes in the story, areas of unexplained genetic variation and of almost symbiotic human reliance by the organism in the face of repeated environmental stress. It chooses (if only in an anthropomorphic sense) not to mutate towards drug resistance and yet it stubbornly defies *in vitro* culture outside of a rabbit, a primate or a human. Its external antigenic protein presentation is so sparse it hardly evokes much lethal immunity. Its internal gene wiring, (its genome), is so puny that it can only encode a few metabolic proteins. This anaemic combination provoked the American biologist Lynn Margulis (1938–2011) to postulate that HIV-AIDS itself was nothing more than the organism responsible for Syphilis fusing its genetic payload with that of its host human cell so as to be completely undetectable. This theory gained little credence, however, even though it was a transmuted expression of her previously highly lauded work on endosymbiosis, the idea that small subcellular structures like the mitochondria were bacteria that our own mammalian cells had long ago absorbed and made their own. Well all of this was quite enough to have me chasing my tail. But it left me sufficiently intrigued not just with the scientific mechanics of Syphilis but also with its impact on an unsuspecting or compliant host. I do not, in this book, aim to master or explain the ancestral codons of this disease but rather to see how its presence impinged on society. Not how it works but instead, the damage it does.

I am in this endeavour much indebted to my publisher Springer-Verlag and to my tireless and patient executive editor Melissa Morton with whom I have worked for now some 20 years. No idea for her is too outlandish, no project something to be shelved. For her tolerance and enthusiasm, I am always grateful. I offer my thanks also to my friend and mentor Professor Riccardo Audisio with whom I have academically worked for the last 30 years and who actively supported the publication of this book. I am most grateful to Dr. Adam Jenney for his insightful and thought-provoking foreword. I would also like to thank Claudia Corti the Curator of the Anatomical Wax Collection at the *Museo di Storia Naturale* in Florence for spending the time with me to examine these marvellous wax models and to show me how they became surrogates for anatomical study when access to real bodies was scarce or even prohibited.

Also my thanks to Thomas Cleerebaut the Curator of the Collection at the Félicien Rops Museum in Namur Belgium for kindly providing me with a reproduction of *La Faucheuse* as Rops' *Mors Syphilitica*. It is a grim reminder of what awaited those who transgressed the boundaries of fidelity and who brazenly wandered the dark *fin-de-siècle* metropolitan alleyways. My thanks also to Ranger Shirley Baxter at the Tuskegee Institute National Historic Site and to Dana Chandler the University Archivist, Tuskegee for kindly providing an image of the John A. Andrew Hospital in Alabama. Appreciation as well to the Lasker Foundation New York which provided a photo of Dr. John Mahoney and for permission to use images from the Fogg Art Museum (Harvard Art Museums), the National Gallery of Washington D.C., the Barnes Foundation Philadelphia, the Metropolitan Museum New York and the British Library. Special thanks also go to Ulricke Fladerer at the Stadel Museum Frankfurt am Main for digital image assistance and to the Wellcome Collection librarians Edward Bishop and Crestina Forcina for their help and support.

Melbourne, Australia   Andrew P. Zbar, M.D. (Lond)., M.B.B.S.,
March 2022   F.R.C.S. (Ed)., F.R.A.C.S., F.S.I.C.C.R (Hon)

Contents

Chapter 1
Announcing the Disease: A Brief Chronology of Syphilitic Events

Abstract For three hundred years after it was first systematically recorded in Europe Syphilis wreaked havoc, rumbling along through generations of the congenitally infected, a lethal and disfiguring disease without cure. Essentially unmanageable the history of the complaint was more a history of its social journey. By the time of the First World War it showed its sensitivity to an arsenical compound Salvarsan which when shipped to the troops locked in the trenches of the front lines was believed to be the last best hope for humanity. As Penicillin made its way to the troops in the Second World War, Syphilis had been controlled but not defeated, transformed from a medieval scourge into a prosaic irritation.

The microbe responsible for Syphilis was only discovered in 1905, a spiriliform bacillus (the spirochaete as it was called) flexing and bending raucously under the microscope and lurking in the purulent fluid derived from a genital ulcer. Only after that could the chemistry of its destruction begin to be developed and with the advent of Penicillin in the 1940s Syphilis became transformed from a disfiguring chronic ailment to a sexualized embarrassment. But its story is far more complex than this. Before it was identified, it had spawned the respectable medical discipline of Syphilology with experts in France and England pontificating on its myriad clinical manifestations and doling out salves and mercury rubs, some legitimate and many the province of quacks.

The recognition of disease became almost an art form with the small bacterium lodging in the brain and ushering in the most bizarre and memorable presentations of behaviour combining grandiose delusions with a timid obsequiousness. The lunatic asylums were replete with Queens of Sheba and wise King Solomons imperiously certain of their domains who at one and the same time might claim command over all the world's languages or to possess the secrets of life but who would sit for hours meekly unraveling wicker baskets. For some like the French novelist Guy de Maupassant (1850–1893), he became its captive doomed to wander the streets of Paris incoherent and incontinent. It would be an ignominious end to a man convinced that his Syphilis had ignited his genius and guided his hand to write complete stories unamended in a single night. The rash of Syphilitic patients in the asylum wards at the *fin-de-siècle* came and went before the appearance of chemically effective treatments, perhaps as some unseen microbial mutation to perceived environmental stress.

In the story of Syphilis, there are many parallels between its emergence and that of HIV/AIDS in the 1980s, not least the vilification of its sufferers and their quarantine from a society built on fear and the threat of contagion. Some like the biologist Stephen Jay Gould (1941–2002) had anticipated an unenviable holocaust from which only the strongest would survive to repopulate the earth. Other's like Susan Sontag (1933–2004) had more soberly foretold that with medical advance and focus that the conquest of AIDS would result in its "de-dramatisation"[1] and that its spectre would transform to a manageable ailment. Syphilis too, had gone through its phases of excommunication and integrated acceptance but had only done so when its diagnosis and treatment had transcended from sorcery to science.

The greatest fear of Ancien régime France in particular was that their hard-won new enlightenment brought by the celebrated philosophers of the age would be undermined by the proliferation of congenital syphilitics impregnating impressionable and clean young French women. It is hard to imagine today but back then there was a national concern that the profusion of such cases, (the *hérédos* as they were referred to), would destroy the intellectual élite of France. The push to understand the heredofamilial nature of the disease, to define its causative agent and to limit its venereal spread became particularly acute. By 1901, it had engendered the establishment in Paris of the Society of Sanitary and Moral Prevention by one of its leading exponents Jean Alfred Fournier (1832–1914) and in so doing had suddenly co-opted the Syphilis experts as the moral arbiters of the community standard. Syphilis, Fournier believed was a threat to the entire human race and it could only be contained by locking up all the prostitutes, mandating their pelvic examinations, certifying them infected or no and detaining all its victims in the lock hospitals. The response to such a crisis would be to pinion the population under siege.

Today, Syphilis, although a modern ailment lives with one foot in history. Only a few infectious diseases like Tuberculosis, malaria, cholera and the Black Death can make a similar claim. This was Syphilis' harsh competitive terrain and it speaks in part of this different era. Today, (at least in the first world), we think of ourselves as relatively insulated from the ravages of some of the commoner deadly infectious illnesses. Although there is still some current controversy and debate concerning routine infant vaccination, (and certainly a vociferous minority who resist the global push to vaccinate against COVID), most of the childhood infectious diseases like mumps, measles, rubella and whooping cough don't impact young lives because of such programs and the same may be said of other more exotic but equally severe infections including smallpox, yellow fever, rabies and poliomyelitis. The COVID era has ushered in a new reticence towards the acceptance of science and is represented by a stubborn coalition that resists vaccination against this particular

---

[1] Sontag, Susan. *AIDS and its Metaphors*. Farrar, Strauss and Giroux 1989; p. 93.

illness over others in a way that is uniquely politicized. The politics of other viral agents like polio seemed less pervasive, today's resistance prolonging pandemics and inviting the prospect of mutations that no longer show susceptibility to generic manufactured mRNA vaccine skeletons.

But those times were different and comparisons cannot be strictly made. Dickensian England represented one of the greatest of threats to young life in particular, where most of these illnesses including diphtheria, scarlet fever, typhoid, cholera, rheumatic fever and Tuberculosis provided a backdrop to the expected hazards of an infant's existence and where up to one-fifth of children succumbed to one or other infectious ailment before they had reached the age of 2 years. Malnutrition too contributed to an overall susceptibility to illness by the turn of the 19th Century where London recruiters for the Boer War rejected 7 out of every 10 applicants for combat primarily because of their lack of fitness. By 1900 up to 500 people a year were believed to starve to death on London's streets at a time when it was estimated that one out of every 7 children under the age of one year succumbed to either congenital Syphilis or intractable diarrhoea.[2]

It was only after the visualization and identification under the microscope of the spirocahete responsible for Syphilis and with the emphasis on effective antibacterials that attempts to contain it shifted from the mere amelioration of symptoms to bacterial eradication. The idea that all microbial disease could be eliminated by a corresponding antimicrobial agent was the brainchild of Robert Koch (1843–1910) who in the late 1890s had established microbiology as a discrete discipline and who had initiated the first bacterial cultures.[3] It would take his disciple Paul Ehrlich (1854–1915) to find what he called his *Zauberkügel* (his magic bullet), the arsenical compound he had named Salvarsan to control the Syphilitic scourge.[4] When it had been developed in Ehrlich's Frankfurt laboratory, (the 606th compound tried against rabbits inoculated with the Syphilis spirochaete), it was quickly mass produced but because it needed to be injected it was sent to way stations rather than

---

[2] The introduction of public water fountains in London provided clean water eradicating the epidemics of diarrhoea. By 1880, the Metropolitan Drinking Fountain and Cattle Trough Association had constructed 800 drinking fountains throughout the city for public and horse use; an effort which needed the support of local philanthropists such as Baroness Angela Burdett-Coutts (1814–1906) and external benefactors including the first Maharajah of Vizianagaram, Pusapati Vijayarama Gajapati Raju (1897–1922).

[3] Robert Koch (1843–1910) was able to isolate the responsible *Mycobacterium* as the cause of Tuberculosis visualizing it by light microscopy and winning him the 1905 Nobel Prize. He created his sacrosanct 4 'Postulates of Microbiology' still in use today concerning how to identify a microorganism putatively responsible for an infectious disease. These are: (1) The organism found should be present in all cases of the disease; (2) The organism should be able to be isolated from an infected host and then grown in a pure culture; (3) Organisms derived from those pure culture lines should produce the disease in healthy animals and (4) In those infected animals the organism can again be isolated, secondarily cultured and found to be identical to the original isolated organism.

[4] Ehrlich's proposal was an entirely chemical paradigm suggesting that 'alien cells' like bacteria possessed toxins on their surface which might be able to be disarmed by a corresponding chemical anti-toxin. His was the first description of cell surface receptors and ushered in the concept of 'chemotherapy' as a chemical means to treat cancer.

directly to the killing fields of the Great War. Here it was extensively used on the Allied troops fresh from the trenches and equally freshly diagnosed with their venereal complaints.[5]

Syphilis was a disease nominated not in its medical history but in lyrical poetry. The polymath Girolamo Fracastoro had nominally ascribed the festering elements of a hideous new disease to the young shepherd Syphilus who had imperiously offended the God Apollo. The beginnings of the disease are contentious. For most, it had burst into Spain aboard Columbus' ships to rampage through Italy lumbering along with the army of Charles VIII and its traveling contingent of military prostitutes as Charles overcame Naples in 1496. But some paleontologists contest that Syphilis had always existed, mirroring the biblical afflictions of Job and sung in the ancient maladies hidden in the papyri of Ebers and in the Akkadian poem *Gilgamesh* which so emulated the ancient story of Noah and the flood.[6] For others, Syphilis would transform into discrete diseases as a response to its environment and manifest with different form in the sub-Saharan desert, the plains of present-day Botswana and the jungles of Central and South America. Only in the west would it venerealize and become the intimate disease we know today.

Why Syphilis should arrive so catastrophically in Renaissance Europe and manifest as a much more aggressive and deadly pestilential disease than it does today is decidedly unclear. Seemingly, after all but conquering its prey, why should it then metamorphose into a distinctly more insidious, less fatal venereal condition modifying its clinical guise and tempo in accordance with ambient environmental and host conditions? Whilst other microorganisms might seek mechanisms dedicated to the evasion of antibiotic therapies or invoke molecular tricks designed to engender drug resistance, the spirochaete remains loyally susceptible to Penicillin and demonstrates no signs of drug resistance. Despite setting the conditions for its worldwide elimination, however, it persists not through some genetic mutational guile as other resistant bacteria do, but by its cozy almost affectionate need to survive in the warmth of human spaces. It survives then even in the presence of a true *Zauberkügel* because of our behaviour as sexual beings.

The story of its treatment is one that moved from alchemy to toxins some of which were as destructive as the disease itself. Mercury (in one form or another), was still so widely used into the early 20th Century that up to half those treated suffered from its toxicity that manifested in a shaking palsy and an irrepressible timidity which mimicked in some the neural syphilitic disease it was designed to correct. The effectiveness of the mercury friction rub could only be gauged after it had sweated out the very life blood of those to whom it had been administered causing the treated to salivate litres of fluid a day. Horrified, their opponents, the 'anti-mercurialists' swore by the healing properties of the guiacum wood, (a

---

[5] At the end of World War 1 it was estimated that nearly one-fifth of the French forces had contracted venereal disease, about 90% of which was gonorrhoea and 10% Syphilis.

[6] In the poem Gilgamesh builds the walls of Uruk and travels to meet with Utnapishtim upon whose legend was formed the basis of the story of Noah's ark.

sudorific sweat producing West Indian plant only found in Hispañola), or of the medicinal powers of Peruvian bark, the Scandinavian Mezereon Daphne or the Sarsparilla root. Over 65,000 doses of Ehrlich's Compound 606 had been sent out free of charge to participating centres throughout Europe and although highly effective, about one in every thousand so treated had serious complications, resulting in a painful lawsuit that although vindicating Ehrlich's work, broke him as a man. By 1943, the wonder drug Penicillin had been shown to eradicate early Syphilis in 4 young servicemen by researchers at the newly established Venereal Diseases Research Laboratory in Staten Island, New York. Its impact would be seismic and as Ehrlich had done during the Great War with his Salvarsan, Penicillin's co-discoverer Howard Florey would by 1944 organize the manufacture of industrial amounts of the drug in time to protect the US Army at its Normandy D-Day landings. Penicillin would tame but never eliminate Syphilis which would rear up in the first decade of the 21st Century with its largest number of cases in Europe and the United Kingdom since the 1950s.[7]

Syphilis has insinuated itself into drama and novels but not in the manner of the more romantic of illnesses, consumption, whose lingering frailty has been more identifiable and more iconic. Not surprisingly, the struggling consumptive has always evoked greater sympathy than the rotting syphilitic and their tubercular terminal throes will invariably remain more sanitized even as they lie amongst blood-stained sheets. Given the majesty of some of its most visible ulcerations and scars, Syphilis surprisingly has had smaller impact upon painting than might be imagined particularly when visual allegories had shown the way to the penitent masses about how it was expected that they should behave and of the consequences of sinful lives. If the visual impression of Syphilis could be distilled into one man, it would personify in Rembrandt's languid portrayal of his favourite pupil, the congenitally syphilitic Gerard de Lairesse (1641–1711) whose facial features of the disorder are textbook almost 200 years before they would first be described. The pock-marked legacy from nefarious dalliances would fuel the moral intonations to a promiscuous audience that was the hallmark of 18th Century caricatures. But that had virtually disappeared in the posters of bawdy Parisian life as seen in the sweet abandonment of the Moulin Rouge or the Folies Bergère. In these there was seemingly little consequence of unfortunate but dangerous liaisons.

Perhaps it is the sexualization of the illness and the fact that there might be a disproportionate number affected amongst the indigent, but there are numerous examples in the medical literature where those suffering from Syphilis have been experimented upon frequently without either their knowledge or consent. The

---

[7] In the decade between 1997 and 2007, in the United Kingdom the registered number of annual cases of Syphilis has increased by nearly 1200% with satellite outbreaks reported in Bristol, Manchester, Brighton and London amongst both heterosexual men (mainly through involvement with commercial sex workers) and the largest contingent from men having sex with men (the so-called MSM group). Amongst the MSM group, about one-third have HIV co-infection. [Data taken from Michael Rayment and Ann K Sullivan. *He who knows syphilis knows medicine—the return of an old friend.* British Journal of Cardiology April 2011; 18: pp. 56–58].

ethical dimension of Syphilis is overshadowed as a byword by the small town of Tuskegee Alabama where for 40 years more than 400 African American men with known Syphilis were denied the treatment available so that the outcomes of unmanaged disease could be observed in the most dispassionate and callous detachment. As poor and frequently illiterate men of the south, they were watched but never heeded, surveyed but never saved. Theirs was the stereotype of the Black male deemed inferior and more susceptible to the commoner afflictions. A race prejudicially thought more prone to contamination, less responsive to the normal medicaments and according to some destined for extinction.

Syphilis defies the philosophical maxim that *"we do not know things well unless we know them in their beginnings"* for its beginning as we shall shortly discover is still in dispute.

Chapter 2
Fracastoro's Poem and the Origins of Illness

Therefore seeing that contagions vary so much in nature and type and that there are many seeds with fascinating characteristics, contemplate this one too whose origin is heaven. It burst into the air, a disease as marvelous as it was strange. It did not infect the silent creatures of the deep, the swarms of those that swim, nor birds, nor dumb animals wandering in high forests, nor herds of oxen or sheep or herds of horses, but out of all the species, the one that is great through its mind, the human race, and it feeds, pasturing deep within our limbs.

Girolamo Fracastoro 'Syphilis sive morbus Gallicus' 1530

Abstract To the Renaissance doctor, historian and scholar Girolamo Fracastoro goes the acclaim of first calling Syphilis by name if only in an epic poem singling out its earliest sufferer Syphilus. But Fracastoro was also the one who laid suggestion that contagious illnesses might be spread on the air by invisible beings some 300 years before Pasteur and Koch could identify bacteria with their microscopes. As the pestilence spread so widely and with such virulence throughout Europe the debate was whether its origin should be laid at the feet of Columbus who brought it back unknowingly from the New World or whether it was a pre-Columbian disease. What defined its intimate association with humans and how did it genetically acquire its propensity to manifest in different continents as yaws, pinta, bejel and in the folklore of remote villages as far apart as Siberia, sub-Saharan Africa and Tierra del Fuego?

Some diseases conjure up the impression of a distinctiveness through their protean manifestations. Others do so in the stories of the struggle for their cure. And still others in the historical nature of their presumptive origins. For Syphilis, it is all three. Today, it seems as an arcane contagion, horridly transmissible, generated in some dark carnal recess and manufactured in secretive shame. If as some had suggested, the legacy of its passionate acquisition and its prolonged and notoriously toxic treatment was *"two minutes with Venus and two years with mercury,"* the apellation that would describe its genesis would be mired with the chauvinistic separation of warring armies and the perception of one's enemies. It was more than

A. P. Zbar, *Syphilis*, https://doi.org/10.1007/978-3-031-08968-8_2

the impression of the causative agents of its onslaught and its very name came to symbolize everything that we detested about other Nation states.

And so the French (in some desperation) would refer to it as the *Neapolitan disease* or the *Spanish illness* and the Neapolitans and the Spaniards would retort by labelling it the *French Evil* or simply the *Morbus Gallicus*. The Poles called it the *Russian illness* and the Russians the *Polish disease*. The Persians gave it the moniker of the *Turkish pestilence*, the Tahitians the *British disease*, the Indians the *Portuguese complaint* and the Japanese the *Chinese Pox,* the *Cantonese ulcer* and the *Tang sore*. Never has a more global ailment found such nominal asylum in the generative bosom of so many nations. Although the actual name, Syphilis itself would be coined by the physician of Verona Girolamo Fracastoro, (1476/8?–1553) most knew of it before he nominally immortalized it in his poem *Syphilus sive morbus Gallicus* in 1530.

As a venereal scourge, its unique and pervasive nature brought it the appellation the *Great Pox* if only to distinguish it from the ancient and highly fatal vesicular smallpox.[1] It had been described before Fracastoro, however, by Jacques de Béthencourt of Rouen as *la Grande Gorre*,[2] with Béthencourt certain of its venereal nature acquired by those engaged in what he thought was the heinous act of copulation with women during their menstrual cycle.[3] But in its appearance, it was initially a mixed disease and the maladies of both Syphilis and gonorrhoea remained inextricably linked. The French physician Thierry de Héry (1505–1599) considered them the same illness of which the most acute of symptoms of gonorrhoea (the *ardeur d'urine* or the *pisse chaude*—the 'hot piss') were just one part. Such was the confusion between these venereally acquired illnesses by the 18th Century, that in an attempt to prove their common origin by a single progenitor (with Syphilis thought wrongly to be the systemic manifestation of localized

---

[1] Smallpox in the 18th Century was a leading cause of death with over 400,000 fatalities in Europe from infection every year. Syphilis became known as 'the Pox' in reference to *les véroles* with Syphilis '*la grosse vérole*' and smallpox '*la petite vérole*'. From its pock-stage Syphilis also became known as *les grosses pocques, le pancque denarre* and *les fievres Saint-Job*. See *Collection des Chronique Nationales Françaises,* vol XLVII *Chroniques de Jean Molinet* by J.-A. Buchon Paris 1828 (vol. 5).

[2] Jacques de Béthencourt. *Nova penitentialis Quadragesima nec non purgatorium in morbum Gallicum, sive Venereum.* Paris 1527. He coined the term 'venereal disease' as homage to its source from "illicit" love. Some places became so infamous for the acquisition and spread of Syphilis that they lent their names to legend. e.g. the *Peste de Bordeaux,* the *mal de Niort,* the *mal du Carrefour de Poitiers,* the *gorre de Rouen.*

[3] The fear of intercourse with menstruating women as a mode of spread for Syphilis had first been suggested by the physician Cataneus. (Jacobi Catanei de Lucamarino) *De Morbo Gallico* Tractatus of 1504.

gonorrhoea), the English surgeon John Hunter (1728–1793) in the most egalitarian fit of experimentation scratched his own skin repeatedly with a barb he had lain in the penile ulcers of his patients, only to soon display the signs of both illnesses. In his journals he states with singularly British detachment that he had delayed his engagement to the coquettish daughter Anne of the genteel society surgeon Robert Home claiming that after a sojourn working as a ship's doctor in the Anglo-French wars on the Belle Isle that he was not sufficiently monied to sustain a relationship. But in truth, it is more likely that he was awaiting a typically slow response to treatment so that at least by the time he had married her he would not be showing the overt signs of both venereal diseases. More than this, it may well be that the irrational outbursts and bombastic personality which had contributed to his European fame as a great teacher may have been partly due to advancing Syphilis of the brain overlaid with the cognitive dissonance induced by the mercury treatments he had self-prescribed and for which London's milliners and cap makers using mercuric nitrate vapours in the felting of animal hides had legitimately attained the sobriquet of "*mad hatters*".[4]

For Héry, even if the basis of Syphilis as a unique bacterial infection remained unknown, the manifestations of all disease could be divined as the most attributable and recognizable imbalances of the bodily humors, (the blood, the phlegm, the yellow and the black bile), artfully described and categorized a millennium and a half before by the Roman physician Galen (129 C.E.–216 C.E.). For any Renaissance physician, it had shown itself most clearly in disturbances of the temperament of those suffering from the disease.[5] Just as the full panoply of its presentations had not yet been completely annotated, nor its causative microorganism even suggested, the only hope was to assuage the dreadful symptoms with a

---

[4] In the 18th Century, Hunter led the 'Unicist' camp that contended that gonorrhoea was just a localized form of Syphilis. The separatists were headed by the Scottish surgeon Benjamin Bell (1749–1806) in his *Treatise on Gonorrhoea virulenta and lues venereal* and the French internist Philippe Ricord (1800–1889). Earlier influential separatist treatises included the *Dissertation medica inauguralis de gonorrhoea virulenta* by Francis Balfour (1767) and Andrew Duncan the Elder's *Observations on the operation and use of Mercury in the Venereal Disease* (1772). Mercury madness such as it was, (referred to as *erethism mercurialis*), was often heralded by uncontrollable tremors. In most cases it resulted in someone who frequently showed a remarkable shyness and unapproachability although in a few cases it caused theatrical outbursts and frank delirium.

[5] The Galenic concept was that all illness represented an imbalance of the 4 basic bodily humors (or vital forces). These included blood, (αἷμα, *haima*) phlegm, (φλέγμα, *phlegma*) black bile (μέλαινα χολή, *melaina chole*) and yellow bile (χολή, *chole*) where disturbances of each would translate into specific temperaments including the sanguine, phlegmatic, choleric and melancholic. [Thierry de Héry. *La méthode curatoire de la maladie vénerienne vulgairment appelée gross variolle et de la diversite de ses symptômes* Paris 1552].

decoction of the bark from a Guaiac tree; a plant which only grew in the New World's Hispañola. Accompanied treatments would then sweat out the illness swaddled in heated blankets that had been saturated in mercurial ointment wrapped around the body in what was called the 'friction method' and for best effect, a recommended placement of a ligation string tightly around the base of the penis.[6]

Regardless of the ghastly tales of its appearance and of the salves and medicaments needed to ameliorate its most foetid symptoms, its name Syphilis, the most recognizable of its elements, can be pinned down to one man, Fracastoro whose lengthy poem would nominally cement it into the lexicon. Fracastoro's lyrical rendition of its symptoms and its treatment with the extracts of exotic plants sang of the great trials those afflicted would endure for a semblance of successful care and of the singular bravery of those willing to venture across the known world in search of both undiscovered territories and remedies.[7] Even if one can argue as to its originality, Fracastoro had borrowed in his symbolism from the writings of the historian Gonzalo Hernandez de Oviedo y Valdez (1478–1557) and most likely fused them to the Roman poet Ovid's opus the *Metamorphoses*.[8] In it, Fracastoro tells the salutary story of the shepherd Syphilus, a man so arrogant that when his land was affected by unremitting drought scolded the Sun God, only to be repaid with a pestilential scourge.[9] It was so personified (manacled to the name of one man), that Syphilus himself became the disease and vice versa.

More than this, Fracastoro marked himself 300 years before the microbiologists Pasteur and Koch could attribute the cause of infectious disease to the transfer and destructive influence of the tiniest microorganisms by his speculative work the *De*

---

[6] The recommendation to use mercurial ointments as a frictional treatment was originally made by (Petrus) Maynardus, Benedictus (Rinius) and Jacobus Cataneus (de Lacu Marcino) at the commencement of the 16th Century along with ligature of the area of any primary syphilitic ulceration which for men meant the usual commencement site of entry—the penis.

[7] Before Fracastoro, Sebastian Brandt wrote of a Syphilis-like illness in his 1496 poem *De pestilentiali Scorra sive mala de Franzos*. Giovanni di Vigo, (Pope Julius II's personal physician) also wrote in his *De Morbo Gallicus* (1514) of a pestilence with such a contagious nature related to sexual intercourse, describing almost perfectly the primary genital ulcers, the short incubation period between this preliminary stage and the secondary rash stage along with the delayed manifestations of chronic syphilitic infection. Much of Valdez' writing widely read in Spanish, English and French editions (*La historia general y natural de las Indias* and *Las Quinquagenas de la nobleza de España*) outlining his experiences in the Indies after 5 New World expeditions has been, however, suggested to have been fabricated.

[8] The Roman poet Ovid (Publius Ovidus Naso) (43 BC–AD 17/18?) constructed his *Metamorphoses* as a chronicle of the history of the world from Creation to the time of the investiture of Julius Caesar as Emperor and his assassination, inspiring the tales of Dante, Boccaccio, Chaucer and Shakespeare.

[9] In the poem in his arrogance, Syphilus convinced the people that the Gods no longer required sacrificial offerings and the King (Alcithous) felt so confident as to declare himself to be a God. When the new disease landed upon the earth in retribution, Syphilus would become its first victim.

contagionibus et contagiosus morbis (the *Treatise on Contagion*) in 1546.[10] Fracastoro postulated the presence of as yet unidentified and unseen particles moving in the polluted air or with the touch that could (he described) spread themselves endemically or rise up intermittently in sine waves of epidemic outbreaks in a manner he explained centuries before bacteria would be discovered or their propensity for the differential patterns of contagious spread would become universally understood.[11] On reflection of his work, it was one of the earliest explanations of the idea of contagion and it occupied his mind particularly during outbreaks of plague like that in Venice in 1534.[12] In it he opposed the idea of infection as part of an atmospheric miasma but more that it could spread directly by the touch, indirectly upon vehicles (which he called the *fomes* or *fomites*) or at distance. Those 'things' that could transmit infection were what he called the *seminaria* or the 'seeds of disease' and these he thought were capable of escalating formally into an epidemic of plague when they landed on putrefying tissue in a susceptible host. It was really the first time that the idea of an epidemic had been analyzed and it challenged the concept that pestilence was a result of God's retribution and that its outcome was therefore immutable.[13] If God could sew the seed, for Fracastoro at least, Man still had control over the soil.

---

[10] Robert Koch (1843–1910) was the pioneer of laboratory bacterial culture. Louis Pasteur (1822–1895) was the proponent of the Germ Theory after he disproved the doctrine of spontaneous generation where microorganisms were incapable of growth in uncontaminated environments. Both established microbiology as a discipline towards the end of the 19th Century.

[11] Fracastoro also described similar patterns of illness for Tuberculosis, Rabies and Measles. [See Hieronymus Fracastorus Veronesis. *Veronesis Opera Omnia.* Venice Junta 154: 77–8].

[12] The notion of contagion was unknown in antiquity and it has no recognizable Greek descriptive word.

[13] Thucydides (460 BC–395 BC) the Athenian historian and General, was perhaps the first to actually suggest that illness might spread from person to person writing of the plague of Athens and influencing other Roman writers on the subject including Livy, Ovid, Pliny the Elder and Seneca. Miasmas (unpleasant or unhealthy vapours in the air) were suggested as the cause of plague in the works of Hippocrates and Lucretius and also in Marcus Aurelius' *Meditations* (Book IX). Divine wrath was thought to control the outcome of epidemics which in suitable cases with prayer might be ameliorated with medication. According to Camerarius "*In times of plague, one's first duty is public penance and then one's medical intervention might prosper*". [From *De recta et necessaria ratione preservandi in pestis contagio*" a synopsis of Girolamo Donzellini, Giovanni Filippo Ingrassi and Cesare Runio: *The Synopsis quorundum...commentariorum de peste.* Nuremberg Garlachi & Montanus 1583]. So too did the Arabic medical literature suggest that plague was the prerogative of Allah as articulated in the *Book of the Pest* by al-Bokhari (810–870 AD) which extensively debates whether Allah actually concerned himself with such trivialities. Contagion however in other illness like leprosy had already been recognized by the Arabic physician Ibn-Zuhr (Avenzoar 1094–162) who suggested that it was transmitted either by '*nearness to lepers or intercourse with them*'. For Fracastoro, Syphilis was the ultimate penitential paradox. Only those receptive and reverent enough not to ever develop the illness in the first place could be exposed to such putrid and evanescent miasmas placing them at risk.

If Fracastoro had made only this single contribution then that alone might be sufficient to include him as Master physician within the pantheon of healers. But there is considerable debate concerning his other scientific achievements particularly in the fields of astronomy and optics and he pre-emptively stands on the definitional boundary of the new science. In his *History of Western Philosophy* Bertrand Russell (1872–1970) separates the period around 1700 as that demarcating the emergence of science.[14] The watershed was probably the introduction by William Harvey (1578–1657) of his new experimental method which posited simple small hypotheses confirmed or refuted by discrete experimentation and which so elegantly described the mechanics of the circulation and the bloodstream and linked them with the rhythmic contractions of the heart. Harvey had first displayed it to a critical audience in the *Theatrum Anatomia* in Padua when he showered the front row with a bloody pulsation after cutting the aorta of a restrained dog in 1628.

In Fracastoro's time science as a distinct discipline did not for all intents and purposes exist. Natural phenomena like eclipses and lightning were considered as portents and omens and the new illnesses whose symptoms he so dutifully recorded were most assuredly the consequence of Divine retribution over sinful lives. Diseases had no specific link to causative agents and their effect and treatments (such as they were), reflected a Godly vengeance which could only be managed rather than simply treated with nothing more than the sacrificial homage to an angered Deity. It was a time of sorcery with battlelines clearly drawn between penitent men and those driven by occult Satanic forces. The prevailing art and literature openly displayed the *ars moriendi* (the art of dying) as much as the *modus vivendi* (the way of living) which would be rewarded with eternal life. The prevailing salves and medicaments for the principal afflictions were designed to restore some Universal harmony to unseen but pervasive humors governing one's underlying personality and well-being. After 1700, such talk of magic found less force in a world whose populace had been shown the elegant symmetry of physical laws to which everything showed obedience. The labours of Galileo, Kepler and Newton to enunciate the new rules of behavior controlling even the movement of the celestial bodies ushered in a modern science where reference to underlying evil forces left the natural phenomena less room to be influenced by the whims of chance. It had paved the way for medicine too to better define the genesis of the common afflictions as having discrete causes which could be treated in their own right and which were divorced from some grander cosmic plan.

---

[14] Bertrand Russell. *The History of Western Philosophy*. Unwin Publishers London 1979 (1946 First Edn): p. 514.

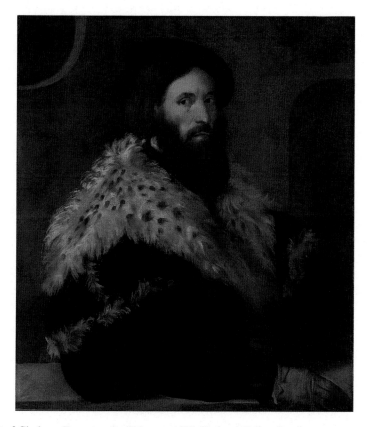

Portrait of Girolamo Fracastoro by Titian *ca.* 1528. National Gallery London

But where did this Fracastoro come from? It is in the affairs of such men, often a measure of their historical importance not only through analysis of their own impact but by defining the company they have kept. One will influence the other and it is apposite to examine Fracastoro by those he knew. His publication the *Syphilus sive morbus Gallicus* was dedicated to his close friend Pietro Bembo, (1470–1547) a man who rose from the most humble (and even primitive) of beginnings to become the administrator of the Diocese of Bergamo and Gubbio, thence a cardinal and ultimately secretary to Pope Leo X.[15] Bembo spent his life (as did Fracastoro), surrounded by books, fancying himself a poet on par with the great Petrarch or

---

[15] Publication of *Syphilus sive morbus Gallicus* was by the da Subbio brothers whose principal interest was in the printing of Greek texts in Latin.

capable in his *Gli Aselani* of writing such prose that would rival that of the legendary Boccaccio. Like the Florentine poet Dante Alighieri too, Bembo devoted large energy to promoting the use in the schools as much as in the streets of the Italian vernacular (the *Prose della vulgar lingua*) and he had himself been greatly influenced by his father Bernardo's pressure on the Council elders of Ravenna to erect a statue of Dante in his honor. Sending his manuscript first to Bembo before its publisher reflected Fracastoro's need for official approval and Bembo in his position felt sufficiently confident so as to insist on over 100 revisions and annotations to Fracastoro's poem before its publication. Changes were made without rancour but some have even argued that they were more than substantive with Bembo's revision made almost to the point of rewriting it himself.

Fracastoro was particularly well connected. He knew the German artist and engraver Albrecht Dürer (1471–1528) and also the theologian Desiderius Erasmus (1466–1536) both of whom also knew Bembo, and he was friends with the artist Raphael (1487–1520).[16] Even as Fracastoro's move from Verona to the idyllic surroundings of Incaffi near the Monte Baldo mountain range was initially designed to escape an outbreak of the plague in 1510, the choice seemed inspired.[17] Incaffi transformed rapidly under Fracastoro's direction into a meeting colony for intellectuals like Ludovico Nogarola (1490?/91–1558) who used it as his vantage point to speculate in his *Timotheus de Nilo* on the contentious source of the river Nile and also to write an epistle for the Roman Catholic Church on Henry VIII's recent divorce to Catharine of Aragon.[18] So too did the noble and connected della Torre family frequent, to visit with Fracastoro. One of them was the young *wunderkind* Professor of Anatomy at Padova, MarcAntonio who had taught Leonardo da Vinci the rudiments of cadaveric dissection in his quest to portray the perfect human form.[19] Another was his brother Giambattista (della Torre) who had stimulated in Fracastoro an abiding love of astronomy.

It was also completely natural to Fracastoro for the rise and fall of serious illness to follow the planetary appositions or the lunar tides and his notions of these epidemics would have found part of their genesis in his astrological charts and in the writings of the young astronomer Nicolas Copernicus (1473–1543). Copernicus too became a friend as well as a student of Fracastoro after entering Padua's medical school in 1501.

---

[16] Fracastoro particularly cherished Erasmus' treatise *On Civility in Children*. Erasmus was a founder of the Collegium Trilingue at the University of Leuven which promoted the study of Latin, Greek and Hebrew so that the ancient texts could be properly interpreted. Bembo also knew the notorious Lucrezia Borgia and was rumored to have been one of her lovers.

[17] See G. Manara. *Interno alla casa di Giordano Fracastoro nella terra d'Incaffi*. Verona 1842.

[18] Ludovici Nogarolae Com. *Veronensis disputation super, Reginae Brittanorum divortio* 1532.

[19] It had been the stated aim of MarcAntonio della Torre (1481–1510) to produce an anatomical treatise with Leonardo but della Torre died prematurely from the plague in 1510 at the age of 30. His brother Giambattista della Torre, an accomplished astronomer who influenced Fracastoro's book the *Homocentrica* also died at a young age from the plague. Fracastoro's *Contagionibus* was dedicated to Giambattista.

As Copernicus' tutor, Fracastoro already held the Chair of Logic and was soon to be appointed the Faculty of Anatomy's *conciliarius anatomicus*.[20] Even though he knew nothing of gravitational pull, Fracastoro was at least cognisant of the laws of attraction and repulsion between inanimate objects (although he failed to articulate them) and he was convinced that each of the planets possessed an independent mind and soul. Such were the times that students influenced Masters sometimes more than the other way around and he became heavily swayed in writing his own *Homocentrica* outlining the structure of the Universe by the Copernican view of the cosmos, borrowing much from Copernicus' *De revolutionibus orbium coelestium* which had proposed an heliocentric universe. The astrological theory on the origins of Syphilis became so established that the Nuremberg artist Albrecht Dürer immortalized its beginnings in his woodcut *The Syphilitic Man* showing a pox-afflicted knight dressed in the garb of the Northern German mercenaries, (the *Landknechten*) as the causative vectors of the spread of disease throughout Germany. Covered in pustules, vesicles and abstemes, the poor knight suffers under an indifferent zodiac with an infelicitous alignment of Saturn, Jupiter and Mars and a stamping of the year 1484 on the woodcut, the year the planets enjoined.[21]

Even though he would adopt the new astronomy to explain the epidemics, Fracastoro positioned himself in the middle ground between Ptolemy's geocentric astronomy and that of his young heretical Polish student, Copernicus.[22] Up until then, Ptolemy had dominated debate concerning the conceptual universe where in his *Almagest* and his *Planetary Hypotheses* the planets revolved around a stationary earth compelling all other heavenly bodies to traverse perfect circles in their trajectories. A partly successful solution had accounted for the slight differences noted in their movements with the need to create eccentric apogees and perigees in their orbits and to attribute small epicycles for each of the planets which necessitated that they spin counter to the main orbit around the earth. Such a complex system was needed to explain why some planets might appear to arrive at points faster and some slower than expected, even giving the occasional impression of retrograde movement. Copernicus by contrast, had advocated 8 spheres for the Universe with a fixed central sun where the most distant sphere was populated by the fixed stars. His revolutionary idea proposed that the appearance of the sun and stars moving around the earth was in fact the result of the earth's rotation on its own axis. Even these modifications could not adequately explain their observed movements and in an

---

[20] Fracastoro was never, however, appointed Professor of Anatomy at Padua.

[21] This unique planetary alignment was thought to have occurred on November 25th 1484 marking the beginnings of European Syphilis. The woodcut is entitled *Vaticinium in Epidemicam Scabiem* but was renamed *The Syphilitic*.

[22] Copernicus was wary about publishing his theories and they were only printed shortly after his death. The idea that the existing Ptolemaic astronomy could be questioned was almost heretical and it would necessitate Galileo's recanting of his findings in 1632 under the impress of the Inquisition. Although Galileo defended his views in his *Dialogue Concerning the Two Chief World Systems* the fact that they appeared so at odds with those of his mentor Pope Urban VIII resulted in Galileo's permanent house arrest.

attempt to reconcile the measurements Fracastoro discarded the small perfect epicycles of the planets. He was unable however, to make the leap of Johannes Kepler some hundred years later that the planets traversed discrete ellipses rather than circles. Without this epiphany and paradigmatic shift Newton too would have been less likely to have understood the differential effect close and far distances had upon planetary movements and the impact gravitational pull could have imposed.

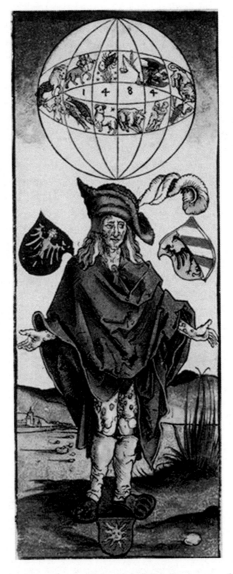

Albrecht Dürer 1496. The woodcut was the illustration for a poem by the Nuremberg city physician Theodoricus Ulsenius, the Vaticinium in epidemicam scabiem

2 Fracastoro's Poem and the Origins of Illness

With the discovery of new continents and isolated in his rural home, Fracastoro's worldview could only become revised through his friendship with navigators and geographers and with the tales they provided of the exploits of other men. One such was Giambattista Ramusio (1485–1557) who faithfully recorded (although with great embellishment) the recent travels of Columbus to the new Americas and Fracastoro would have readily devoured Ramusio's *Navigazione et Viaggi* (Navigations and Travels) whose 3 volumes published just up the road in Venice had even excitedly told of the architectural detail of the legendary city of Atlantis.[23] Such was Fracastoro's world that spawned his morbid tale of the plights of Syphilus but it was also a world that revered his poetry and his prophecy.

Today, if you walk through the Piazza dei Signori in Verona it is dominated by a statue of the poet Dante sculpted by Ugo Zannoni (1836–1919) in 1865. Looking behind and lifting your eyes above an archway is a smaller far less obtrusive statue of Girolamo Fracastoro which was sculpted by Danese Cattaneo (1512–1572) in 1559. Fracastoro is holding the orb of the earth in his right hand and legend tells that the orb will fall if only one honorable man walks under the arch. So far it has remained firmly in his hand.

---

[23] Ramusio's work spanned the cartography of the Old and the developing New Worlds. The book also contained fictionalized accounts of the travels of legendary explorers including Marco Polo, Niccolò Da Conti (who had travelled to India in the early 15th Century), Ferdinand Magellan, Alvar Nuñez Cabeza de Vaca (a Sevillan New World explorer who had lived amongst the exotic Native American Indian tribes in the 1530s) and of Giosafat Barbaro's extraordinary expedition to Persia and the Tartary region of northern central Asia stretching from the Caspian Sea to the Urals and across the current day Caucasus, Siberia and Mongolia. De Vaca's 1555 *La relacion y comentarios del gouernador* relayed his trip to Emperor Charles V to "*transmit what I saw and heard in the ...[years] I wandered lost and miserable over many remote lands*". Barbaro had published his account in the "*Viaggi falti da Venezia alla Tana in Persi*" between 1543 and 1545. Manutius publishers. [See *Travels to Tana and Persia* by Giosafat Barbaro and Ambrogio Contarini, 1494].

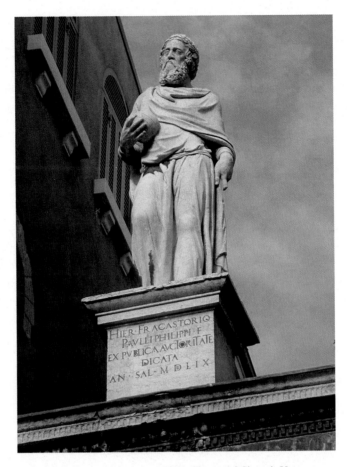

Statue of Girolamo Fracastoro by Cattaneo (1559). Piazza dei Signori, Verona

Even if we can agree about the beginnings of its name and of those who wrote of its manner of spread, it does not dispel the debate concerning the origins of the disease in Europe or even if it is one type of disorder. Renaissance physicians wrote extensively of the risks of 'impure coitus' but the fears of its contagion might mirror those which appeared at the beginnings of HIV-AIDS in the 1980s. The physician Antonio Musa Brassavoli (1500–1555) who tended the Kings Francis I, Charles V and Henry VIII went around warning in particular of its spread through kissing (*oscula cum vibratione et conflictu linguarum*).[24] But the true origins of the illness remain in dispute even today. Most believe it to be what one might call 'a Columbian disease' abruptly appearing in devastating fashion somewhere around 1493 with the arrival of the first ships returning from the New Americas and hence

---

[24] Antonii Musae Brassavoli *Ferrarensis de morbo Gallico* 1551.

with the crews of the Admiral Christoforo Columbus.[25] By contrast, the 'Pre-Columbian' theory would suggest that it was a disorder no different from that which had existed in the Old World before Columbus had returned. In this open debate, the Columbians outweigh the pre-Columbians, with the latter unable to produce any unequivocal descriptions of the disease from antiquity. In this, it has been cogently argued that the greatest of physicians of ancient times, Hippocrates, Galen and Avicenna would in all of their practices have come across something similar and so prevalent and hence within their copious notations would have at least written about the disease. But in all their works, there seems to be nothing on the matter. Even the biblical descriptions of the pestilential trials of Job and his disfiguring ulcerations could not of themselves prove to be descriptions of the same illness. Moreover, with Syphilis producing somewhat classical advanced lesions within the bones in particular, there had never been an observed case of pre-Columbian bones from the Old World which had been unearthed showing unequivocal signs of syphilitic inflammation.[26]

But an absence of something in the literature does not mean that it was never there. First-hand records from those physicians living and working around the ports of call of the returning Genoese ships are testament to the suddenness of the appearance of Syphilis as well as its most devastating 'malignant' presentation upon an unsuspecting public without presumably any prior exposure or immunity. Each records the remarkable rapidity of its European spread. If the disease had been seen before, it most assuredly had not previously appeared either in this form or in this severity. Curiously, however, it never seemed evident to anyone at the time of Columbus' return that they were witnessing something special as an epidemic. This only seemed to occur to people almost two generations afterwards. It was only then too that the guiacum West Indian wood became a popular cure for Syphilis and it would seem inherently logical that both disease and cure should emanate from the same place.[27]

But even if the archeological evidence would favour the Columbian hypothesis, as a theory it has problems fitting the facts. For the Columbian theory to survive, we have to imagine a conspiracy that Columbus would have deliberately omitted the

---

[25] *"In the yere of Chryst 1493 or there aboute……. this most foule and most grievous dysease beganne to sprede amonge the people"* as recorded by Ulrich von Hutten in his *"Of the wood guiacum"*. London Thomas Bertheleltregii 1540.

[26] It has been argued that similar illnesses were described by Pliny the Younger (61–100 AD) and by Paul of Aegina, (625–690 AD) a Byzantine physician who compiled a medical compendium of disease in the 7th Century. The Roman poet Horace (Quintus Horatius Flaccus) (65–8 BC) wrote of a *morbus campanus* (a country malady) with many of the features of secondary Syphilis as did other poets and satirists such as Marcus Valerius Martialis known as Martial (38–41 AD?-102–104 AD?) and Decius Lunius Iuvenalis also known as Juvenal, (55–60 AD?-127 AD). Both had written that the illness they had witnessed was the result of the practice of incessant pederasty.

[27] *"Our lord GOD from whence this evill of the Poxe came, from thence would come the remedy for them"* as quoted in Nicolas Monardes. *"Ioyfull newes out of the New Founde Worlde"*. John Frampton *transl.* London Willyam Norton 1577: 10r. Quoted in *The Early History of Syphilis* by Alfred W. Crosby Jr. *American Anthropologist* 1969; 71: 218–227.

nature of such a severe illness he knew was aboard his ships and further, that that conspiracy would have followed him through Spain and Portugal at all his ports of call where no such illness was found or treated. There was too a clear hiatus between his return and the first reported outbreaks of the contagion in 1494 which would belie its inherently venereal nature. Columbus made sure he was the only chronicler of the voyage (and then after him his son Ferdinand who authored Columbus' biography) but even then it is unlikely that he would not know of the conditions aboard his other ships despite his own Santa Maria losing contact with the Pinta and the Niña after severe storms.[28] Gonzalo Hernandez de Oviedo y Valdez (1478–1557) adamantly blames Columbus for the European epidemic and so too does the Spanish historian and devout Franciscan monk Bartolomeo de Las Casas (1484–1566) who was noted for his strong critiques of Oviedo.

Las Casas became a passionate advocate for the Native Indian and wrote in his *Short Account of the Destruction of the Indies* in 1542 about the atrocities committed against the indigenous natives by the Spanish conquistadors.[29] Las Casas was well placed for commentary. He had been in Seville when Columbus sailed into the city in 1493 and both his father and his uncle were on board the Santa Maria. As for Oviedo, he had already met Columbus prior to his most famous 1492 voyage and knew both of Columbus' sons well. Both Las Casas and Oviedo were also well acquainted with one of the most powerful families, the Pinzóns, a rich merchant group who hailed from Palos de Frontera in the Andalusia and who as amongst the most experienced commercial sailors of the Spanish coast had financed the movement of Spanish armadas against Portugal. Along with King Ferdinand and Queen Isabella, the Pinzón family had shouldered the monetary burden of Columbus' first expedition.[30]

By the time the finest of the three Pinzon brothers, Martin Alonso Pinzón (1441–1493) returned to Spain as Captain of the *Pinta* he was desperately ill. Martin had been strong enough to forestall the mutiny that would have certainly developed when Columbus' sailors had grown restless on the journey without a single sighting of land. He had begged them to wait just three more days before contemplating a

---

[28] His work was instrumental in the passage of the so-called New Laws of 1542, the first European ruling abolishing colonial slavery. It also sparked the Valladolid debates of 1550 which examined the theological response of the Spaniards to New World colonization and its peoples.

[29] Despite an imperative towards Catholic conversion and an abhorrence with native practices (in some countries) of cannibalism, Las Casas was the first to argue that colonial powers had no dominion over native rights.

[30] The other brothers of the Pinzón family travelling with Columbus included Francisco Martín (Master of the ship *Pinta*) and Vicente Yañez Pinzon, captain of the ship *La Niña* who is credited on a later trip with the discovery of Brazil. The Pinzon family reputedly put up half a million Iberian maravedi coins towards the costs of Columbus' first expedition, matching that given by the monarchy.

return to Spain. History would have been very different if not for one of his lowly crew, Rodrigo de Triana (1469–1535) on the Pinta first shouting *Tierra! Tierra!* after sighting the coast of the Americas at 2 am on the 12th October 1492.[31] Pinzón, returning to Spain gravely ill was immediately attended by the Sevillano physician Ruiz Diaz de Isla (1465–70?-1542) who also treated several other ill crew members for fevers and widespread skin lesions. According to da Isla, this was like no other affliction he had previously seen.[32] If such oral testimony is anything to go by, its spread across to Barcelona (somewhat aided by a contingent of Catalan prostitutes) and thence by 1494 to the warring army of afflicted Spaniards which had joined King Charles VIII of France (Charles the Affable) was crucial in conquering the Kingdom of Naples.[33] This temporal association is confused by the conflated arrival with Columbus' sailors of typhus and typhoid fever and by the release of many

---

[31] The site of the first American landfall is debated. Columbus named it San Salvador (and the natives called it Guanahani). It was most likely one of the islands of the Turks and Caicos group. To calm his sailors Columbus had promised that the crew member who first sighted land would receive an annual stipend of 10,000 gold coins for life. When Triana claimed the prize Columbus informed him that he personally had sighted land at 10 pm the night before but did not think it significant enough to inform anyone, claiming the monies for himself. "*It was so indistinct that [1 do] not dare to affirm it was land*" he wrote in his diary (*Esta tierra vidó primero un marinero que se decía Rodrigo de Triana, puesto que el Almirante a las diez de la noche, estando en el castillo de popa, vidó lumbre aunque fue cosa tan cerrada que no quiso afirmar que fuese tierra* .... This land was first seen by a sailor who called himself Rodrigo de Triana, since the Admiral at ten o'clock at night, being in the stern castle, saw fire although it was so closed that he did not want to affirm that it was land). On his return to Spain, Triana converted to Islam with reports that unable to recover, he committed suicide.

[32] Da Isla called the illness the *Morbo Serpentino* in a publication the *Tractado llamado fructo de todos sanctos: contra el mal serpentino* which appeared until 1539. By this stage the skin lesions (the *apostemes*) and enlarged glands (the *bubas*) were equivalent to the Hispañolan abnormalities documented called the *goayaras*, (or *guynaras*) the *hipas*, the *taybas* and the *iças*.

[33] The entry (and the spread) of Syphilis into Italy has variously been blamed on many sources including the sailors who had travelled with Columbus, women he had brought back from the New World, the influx of Jews expelled from Spain under the threat of the Spanish Inquisition for not converting to Christianity, extraneous Spanish troops sent by King Ferdinand to assist King Alphonso II of Naples to repel the French and to the 500 or more prostitutes who had travelled along with King Ferdinand's army. Some even attributed it to fringe Christian sects like the *Brethren of the Free Spirit* whose practice of praying in the nude and promoting sexual freedoms had provoked the ire of Pope Boniface VIII in 1296 and Pope Clement V in 1311. [See Arthur Versluis. *The secret history of Western sexual mysticism: Sacred practices and spiritual marriage* Destiny Books 2008: p. 63]. Like many diseases for which blame is not apparent and where the cause seems occult or unknowable, legend may personalize it with one tale being spread that it had started when a leprous knight had intercourse with a loose courtesan. In another rumour of the times it was suggested that the disease emerged following sexual intercourse between men and monkeys or that Greek wine had been deliberately spiked with leprous blood. Attribution by the English syphilologist Sir Thomas Sydenham (1624–1689) to the African slave trade (via the Americas) could not be correct since British slave movement did not even commence until 1503.

suffering leprosy after Pope Innocent VIII had closed the leprariums and had unsuccessfully tried to merge the Order of St Lazarus with the Sovereign Military Order of Malta in 1489.[34]

Given the debate about the entry of Syphilis into Europe, there are two other points of interest. The first of these can be found in the bones. Paleoanthropologists like Bruce Rothschild from Youngstown and North Eastern Ohio Universities have pointed to the relatively specific osseous legacy of chronic advanced Syphilis that pathologists have known about for years. He and his researchers make distinction between these changes and those that are referred to as taphonomic degeneration (that which occurs after death). Specific bony marks of Syphilis include the curvature of the tibial shinbone of the leg (referred to as the sabre tibia because of its resemblance to a scimitar) and the thickened ridge along the course of the bone that represents a chronic periosteal reaction. So too do children with congenital Syphilis show a characteristic dentition with notched incisor teeth that were first described by the English physician Sir Jonathan Hutchinson (1828–1913) and which are known as 'Hutchinson's teeth'.[35] With these criteria we do not see undisputed cases

[34] St. Lazarus was the patron saint of lepers and the Order of St Lazarus of Jerusalem had been established by crusaders in 1119 specifically to care for them. It had been sanctioned by a Papal Bull issued by Pope Alexander IV in 1255 as *Cum a Nobis petitur*. The closure of many leper colonies forced sufferers into the main cities seeking food and shelter. Traditionally, St. Denis is described as the Patron Saint of syphilitics although the origin of this patronage is debated. The association between Syphilis sufferers and St. Denis has been attributed to Karl Sudhoff's *Graphische und Typographische Erstlinge der Syphilis literatur aus den Jahren 1495–1498* (of 1925) in a quoted poem: "*O most Holy Father and mighty helper. Denis; Archbishop and praiseworthy martyr. ...protect me from the terrible disease called the French malady from which you freed a great many Christian people in France when they tasted the water from the living spring which welled up from beneath your sacred body.*" St. Denis as the first Bishop of Paris had come from Rome in order to convert the population some time between 272 and 290 AD. Following his arrival he was arrested and beheaded with his disciples. Legend reports the miracle that his headless body carried the head over a long distance collapsing finally at the feet of a Christian woman Catulla who buried him there and established an abbey. The story holds more wonder than other tales which say that following his execution his body was simply thrown into the River Seine. Dulaure's *Histoire de Paris* (1821–1825) reports that at least 7 reliquary heads of St. Denis can be found throughout France. [See Dulaure JA. *Histoire de Paris*. Guillaume Paris 1821–1825. See Also Sudhoff K. *The earliest printed literature on Syphilis. Being Ten Tractates from the years 1495–1498*. Adapted by C. Singer Lier Florence. 1925 and *Butler's Lives of the Saints*. H. Thurston and D. Attwater (Eds). Volume 4 2nd Edn. Burnes & Oates London]. The associative link between St. Denis and Syphilis is one of place only and was suggested after Thierry de Héry had remarked to a priest as he knelt before a statue of Charles VIII in the Chapel of St. Denis (in Nôtre Dame) that "*Charles VIII is a good enough Saint for me. He put 30000 Francs in my pocket when he brought the pox to France.*" De Héry had been made rich treating syphilitic soldiers after Charles VIII Italian campaign.

[35] Jonathan Hutchinson (1828–1913) was the first to link peculiarly notched incisor teeth, deafness and interstitial keratitic inflammation of the eyes as hallmarks of congenital Syphilis. The three signs are referred to as Hutchinson's triad.

in the Europe of the Old World although they have been consistently found in the New World predating Columbus' arrival. This strongly suggests that Syphilis was imported on Columbus' return.[36]

The second caveat is the introduction of the Unitarian hypothesis of the origin of Syphilis as proposed in the 1950s by the physician and Syphilis expert Ellis Herndon Hudson (1890–1992). It is not surprising that Hudson posited a socio-logical theory of the origin of Syphilis which he postulated had been present well before Columbus but in different guise, metamorphosing into different types of illness depending upon the climate and the social circumstances of evolving civi-lizations. One might imagine that in its newest form arriving in Europe it might behave like other epidemic illnesses, spreading rapidly with an extreme virulence and ultimately calming its severity after killing off the most vulnerable hosts with the weakest inherent or developed immunity. That would be the mechanism of destruction for a devastating epidemic like the Black Death, but Syphilis according to Hudson became many diseases which produced their own pattern recognition and try as one might in the laboratory to distinguish the different species of bac-terium accounting for each disease type, the microbial culprit seemed identical between the different forms the disease took in different parts of the world. Regardless of which theory one believes, this would imply that the various ailments caused by the same organism occur in different environments rather that that dif-ferent subspecies produce different diseases.

For some reason, the microorganism had settled into a symbiotic relationship with its human host and had stayed there.[37] Only after the microbe would be discovered in syphilitic tissues by specialized microscopy would it be allocated as

---

[36] There has been further dispute concerning the Columbian hypothesis with the discovery of skeletal remains at the ruins of the Blackfriar's monastery in Hull in the United Kingdom showing changes consistent with chronic Syphilis and carbon dating the bones from between 1300 and 1420. The practice of attributing changes in the bones of the Stone Age to Syphilis began in 1877 with the paediatrician Joseph-Marie Jules Parrot (1829–1883) of the Hôpital des Enfants Assistés de Paris who had a specialized interest in hereditary and congenital disease. Rothschild has also linked similar bony changes in personally conducted digs in the Dominican Republic with others, unearthing skeletal remains over 8000 years old in Windover Florida, Frontenac Island New York and Amaknak Island in southwest Alaska suggesting that these changes are due to a non-venereal generic relative of Syphilis. This data would suggest that the changes in the UK skeletons are due to a non-venereal (and hence a different form) of syphilitic-type infection which shows similar changes in the bones. In this respect, isolated cases have been suggested that attempt to refute the Columbian theory including one skeleton from Lisieux in France from the 4th Century AD excavated by Joel Blondiaux and Alduc-Le Bagousse and a similar case from Metaponte in Italy, (6th Century BC), a 12th–14th Century specimen from Poland, one from the 1st Century AD in Agripalle India and another from the Song Dynasty era in China (960–1279 AD). One further possible example of pre-Columbian Syphilis are the remains of the Westphalian knight Gottfried von Cappenberg (1097–1127).

[37] The relationship may not so much be symbiotic as more correctly called amensalistic. In symbiosis a long-term interaction between host and organism is directed towards mutual benefit but in amensalism one organism (in this case the host) can be harmed whilst the other (the bacillus) remains unaffected.

the cause of a range of different diseases. Because of its spiral structure and its complex gymnastic flexural movements it would initially be labelled a spirochaete. Only later would it be renamed into the genus of organisms called *Treponemes* (or *Treponema*) so that Syphilis and its related infections are all examples of a variety of illnesses collectively known as the Treponematoses. But even if we could accept where the *Treponeme* had possibly come from, its origins failed to adequately define its subsequent behaviour.

The story of Syphilis as a distinctly venereal disease is a competitive one. Its disease types reflect this competition and the pattern recognition of its different guises are a measure of its responses to environmental stress. Each illness which we recognize is one of the legion T*reponematoses* which carries its history on its back. The spirochaete is the cause of 4 discrete clinical syndromes; venereal syphilis, non-venereal syphilis, *yaws* and *pinta* and although different subspecies of *Treponemes* have been ascribed to each, there is nothing in the laboratory to distinguish between each subtype. For any bacterium that, it must be conceded, is quite a trick.

And so *Yaws* that once infected 50 million children from sub-Saharan Africa to the southern reaches of Algeria left its visible marks in the depigmented skin and chronic ulcers of its sufferers.[38] It emerged from the hot humid climates of central Africa to penetrate the human body only to lose its genetic trail as an innocuous saprophyte living off decaying skin. It is a disease of childhood preternaturally suited to the close dampness of primitive village life. From there it would move as an endemic Syphilis, the *dischuchwa* of the Bechuanaland bushmen and the *bejel* of the Syrian Bedouins, changing its climate, its custom and its folklore.[39] In this form it manifested as mouth erosions, chronic skin ulcers and a slow forming bone infection spreading to southwestern Asia and up from northern Africa to the Mediterranean basin, finally settling itself into the south Saharan edge, the

---

[38] Yaws (caused by the *T. pertenue* subspecies) is also known as Pian (Fr), framboesia (German, Dutch), buba (Spanish) and bouba (Portuguese). It is a disease of the warm humid regions of Central and South America and the Caribbean as well as tropical Africa and equatorial southeast Asia. It has a 'partner illness' in west African monkeys and baboons. In active Yaws, the initial papule appears as what is called 'a mother yaw' or a 'framboesioma' rich in *Treponemes*. This phase lasts about 3–6 months and heals like a syphilitic chancre with the subsequent development of a secondary phase. In Yaws, like Syphilis there is a relatively non-infectious latency period which can last a lifetime. This may be interrupted at any time by infectious states occurring over 5 yearly intervals.

[39] This non-venereal endemic form of Syphilis (due also to *T. pallidum*) is known throughout the Arabic world as *Bejel* but also in Zimbabwe as *njovera*. It was recognized in the folklore of Europe where in Scotland in the 18th Century it was the *sibbens* and in the coastal towns of Norway it appeared as the *Radesyge*. In Slovenia it was named after the town where it surfaced as an epidemic, the *Skerljevo* most likely affecting the Muslim populations during the military campaign conducted by Mehmet Pasha in 1832. The 1950s saw a similar epidemic in Bosnia–Herzegovina which was controlled under the auspices of the WHO and UNICEF with widespread Penicillin dosing and improvements in local overcrowded housing. [See *Epidemic Syphilis in Bosnia and Studies on the Treponeme: From Causes of Endemic Syphilis*. Bulletin of the World Health Organization 1952].

Sahel.[40] But with the domestication of people throughout Africa and the formation of small societies from nomadic villages and the close order of their housing it had penetrated the orifices of the hunter gatherers in their Asian migration. And then, for some reason, it finally ran out of steam in Brazil, Columbia, Cuba and Mexico moving slowly across the Gulf of Derian in the northwest to Tierra del Fuego in the south as a disease called *Pinta*; a soft ailment and a shadow of its previous incarnations that left only pale depigmented patches on the skin.[41] From there it has venereal cousins across the Siberian tundra and the Alaskan wilderness and towards New Guinea and the Pacific islands where it is the *Irkintja* of the Australian aborigine.[42] Even though these illnesses were all putatively caused by different subspecies, they all appear alike under the microscope and each possesses the same characteristic motility, the same antibody reactivity in the blood and the same genetic backbone. If these transformations and mutations of the syphilitic microorganism are true, why would it relinquish its lethality to become less potent?[43]

Within this new taxonomy of Treponematoses, Syphilis would have a unique history and adaptive evolution. In the way we understand the Hudsonian theory, the bacillus had learned (if a bacterium can so do) to penetrate the human body. But in becoming the Syphilis we understand today, in this endeavour for a belated supremacy it could only enter through the most intimate of means. Even though we understand the nature of the disease today we are unable to interpret either its past incarnations or its distinct character. Like some other infective illnesses, typhus, typhoid, the plague and smallpox, the 'seeds' needed to transform as much as the 'soil' and it had led to the venerealization of the disease.

Even this new theory however, is not enough. It demands that when Syphilis entered Europe with Columbus, that it mutated resulting in the most deadly example of a very old disease.[44] Having then killed its most susceptible victims, it then retreated into a more occult, indolent chronic inflammatory disorder that

---

[40] The Sahel is the climatic transition region between the Sahara (to the north) and the savannah of the Sudan (to the south).

[41] *Pinta* (due to *T. carateum*) is also known in Spain, Argentina, Chile, Peru, Paraguay, Uruguay, Venezuela and Guatemala as the *Azul*, the *Carate*, the *Lota* and the *Empeines*.

[42] It was estimated that after World War 2 that up to 50 million people had Yaws. Between 1950 and 1970, the WHO and UNICEF initiated a global campaign to eradicate it in 46 different countries.

[43] This is a little like the 'dilemma' of HIV infection where in its early years as treatments improved patients began to survive long enough to see some of its more delayed manifestations.

[44] This theory does not account for the conflated idea of horrible disease which may represent different variants of non-venereal ailments like leprosy or venereal examples such as the soft chancre, also called the *Chancroid* which resembles a syphilitic chancre. Chancroid which may reinfect the host is due to another bacterium *Haemophilus Ducreyii*. It is likely that many of these historical diseases were confused (leaving no genetic signature) or that they might have represented a hybrid of illnesses under a range of names including *Arab leprosy*, *elephantiasus Arabum*, the *Great Scab*, *Buvas*, *Mentulagra* and *Venereal leprosy*.

nestled into the bones or in some remained in almost gentle harmony with its host.[45] The contentious nature of the argument between the Columbians (or 'Americanists') and the pre-Columbians (the 'Anti-Americanists') raged with ferocity in the German literature at the turn of the 20th Century. On one side was the chronicler of sexual habits from Lower Saxony Iwan Bloch (1872–1922) who had been an inspiration for Sigmund Freud and who had himself been motivated by what he (i.e. Bloch) had read on the origins of Syphilis from France's men of letters, Montesquieu and Voltaire. Both in their writings had been certain that Columbus had brought the pestilence to Europe.[46] On the other side was Karl Sudhoff, (1853–1938) a medical historian staunchly opposed who in support of his view that Syphilis had been present from time immemorial was the first to examine the signature of Syphilis in the bones disinterred from the necropoli of his home town Leipzig. Syphilis then stands at the crossroads of history. Whichever theory we adopt defines what we are to make of Admiral Don Christopher Columbus. Either he stands with Marco Polo perhaps as the greatest example known of an explorer who brought a new vision to our world consciousness or he unwittingly falls amongst the greatest villains recorded in human history.

---

[45] This would mirror the words of Oviedo *"the bubas comes from the Indes where it is very common amongst the Indians, but not so dangerous in those lands as it is in our own"*. [In Gonzalo Fernandez de Oviedo y Valdez. *La historia general de las Indias.* Seville 1535/Vallodolid 1537]. The idea that Syphilis predated Columbus but that somehow upon entry to Europe it *"acquired a fermentative virulence"* had been proposed well before Ellis Hudson had suggested his Unitarian hypothesis by the Neapolitan physician Charles Musitano in 1711 in his *Traité de la maladie vénérienne.* [See also Laura J. McGough. Gender, Sexuality and Syphilis in Early Modern Venice. The disease that came to stay. Ed Rab Houst and Edward Muir. Palgrave MacMillan 2010].

[46] The French writer Montesquieu, [Charles-Louis de Secondat (1689–1755)] had described the connection between Columbus and the sudden emergence of Syphilis in Europe in his *L'esprit des lois* in 1748 as had Voltaire, [Francois-Marie Arouet (1694–1778)] in his *L'homme aux quarante écus* in 1768.

Chapter 3
The Protean Manifestations of Disease

It was true indeed that I had got the sickness; but I believe I caught it from that fine young servant-girl whom I was keeping when my house was robbed. The French disease; for it was that, remained in me for more than four months dormant before it showed itself, and then it broke out on my whole body at one instant. I went on treating myself according to their (the doctors') methods, but derived no benefit. At last, then, I resolved on taking the wood (guiac) against the advice of the first physician in Rome, and after a few days, I perceived in me great amendment....at the end of fifty days I was cured and as sound as a fish in water.
Benvenuto Cellini (1500–1571)
Florentine sculptor and goldsmith

Abstract The disease inflicts itself on the patient incrementally in stages. First is the small often painless chancre, usually a transient hallmark somewhere (but certainly not always) on the genitalia. It may in women be hidden and remain undiagnosed. A few months later is a second highly contagious secondary stage marked by cutaneous syphylides presenting as a scaly elevated papular rash which includes the palms and soles and where there is often extensive mouth ulceration. Years later, the patient may enter a tertiary stage marked by deep seated abscesses (called *gummata*) which can be located anywhere in the body mimicking cancers in these locales. In the late 19th Century the asylums were filled with neurosyphilitics who presented with discrete disorders of the spinal cord (*tabes dorsalis*) and a remarkable presentation of madness (*General Paresis of the Insane*). The other social impact was the group of congenital syphylitics who grew up as what the French called the *hérédos* and who were thought the greatest risk of infecting the élite intelligentsia.

Even when the earliest descriptions of the 'Great Pox' seemed unusually brutal, 19th Century reports of the disease (which appeared mild by comparison to the Renaissance scourge), proved sufficiently frightening for most. Syphilis was unique, relaying itself in different stages each if untreated, more devastating than its predecessor. It lay dormant for prolonged latent periods, finally to fester in the bones and in the central nervous system in a manner which permitted it bizarre guises and it possessed a legendary capacity to mimic other chronic and seemingly untreatable ailments. Its occult nature and surreptitious insinuation into almost all organ systems proved one of its most effective strategies negating its own treatment. By virtue of its chronicity it became a master of confusion with some symptoms so subtle as to escape routine detection and others so physically and mentally waring that they would become iconic.[1]

In its simplest and most recognizably hateful form it would follow the description by Ulrich von Hutten (1488–1523) that had latched itself like a limpet to Fracastoro's poem with *"byles, sharpe and standing out, havying the similitude and quantite of acornes, from which came so foule humours, and so great stenche, that who so ever one smelled it, thought hym selfe to be enfect"*.[2] It was an abomination implicating all the bodily senses. None would know of its mechanism of spread and all would fear the penetrating corrupted miasmas that drew it across a defilement of the breathable air (the *inquinamenta aeris*).[3] In her book *Illness as Metaphor*, Susan Sontag defines the way that Tuberculosis has been superseded by cancer as the disease of the social age and in it she describes how consumption 'gallops' but cancer with its 'stages' has no apparent gait.[4] So too can the tempo of syphilitic infection be its defining character, sometimes almost malignant in its style, occult and insidious. Protective of its own mantle and mimicking other diseases like a butcherbird, it became the 'great imitator' moving sinuously and sufficiently slowly between its incarnations.[5]

It thrived also (in an era when there was little effective treatment), upon a secrecy in its diagnosis even when its inexorable signs would in many become glaringly obvious. The French novelist and *bon vivant* Gustave Flaubert (1821–1880) commented in a folio of disparate papers he entitled his *Dictionary of Accepted Ideas* that Syphilis was *"as common as the cold.... more or less everybody is affected by it"*.[6] But although he wrote in 1856 in almost obsessive detail to his friend the dramatist Louis Bouilhet (1822–1869) about each minor bodily complaint and corruption, he was still reticent to call his illness by name.[7] The

---

[1] B. Cellini (1500–1571). *The Life of Benvenuto, Son of Master Giovanni Cellini, the Florentine. Written by himself in Florence.* 2 vols. The Navarre Society London 1927 Edn. The first printed edition of this incomplete work appeared in 1728 and was not widely known outside Italy until the beginning of the 19th Century.

[2] Ulrich von Hutten. *Of the wood called guiacaum.* London Thomas Bertehelentregii. 1540.

[3] Fracastoro's theory of contagion would battle with that of his greatest rival the Veronese physician Giovanni Battista Da Monte (1498–1551) that pestilence was vapourously carried in the air. The 'miasma' theory was also promoted by the Breslau physician Johann Crato von Crafftheim (1519–1585) who thought pestilential airs the principal agents of the spread of Bubonic plague.

[4] Susan Sontag. *Illness as Metaphor.* 1978. Farrar, Strauss and Giroux New York, pp. 13, 14.

[5] The British syphilologist, Sir Jonathan Hutchinson wrote of Syphilis that *"All the various phenomena of disease due to syphilis are imitations of other, non-specific type forms ... We have absolutely no malady which is peculiar to syphilis"*. J Hutchinson, *Syphilis* (London, Paris, New York: Cassell & Co, 1887), p. 485.

[6] Flaubert's notes of the 1870s were collated between 1911 and 1913. Vol. 1: pp. 304, 306.

[7] See *The Letters of Gustave Flaubert (1830–1857).* G. Flaubert and Francis Steegmuller. Bellknap Press 1980.

transformation too of Lord Randolph Henry Spencer-Churchill (1849–1895) from a Tory rising star of the British establishment in the 1880s to an incoherent trembling mess unable to deliver his parliamentary addresses might have been labelled by his physician Dr. Thomas Buzzard (1831–1919) as 'general paresis' but the good doctor never felt compelled to treat Randolph with mercurials or any other medication likely to impede that particular diagnosis.[8]

Perhaps the first to recognize that Syphilis had stages of clinical presentation was Juan de Vigo (1450–1525) a surgeon travelling with Pope Julius II. de Vigo noted its orderly progression from a primary ulcer, through to a secondary stage dominated by painful skin papules and from there a latency or dormancy before erupting again as deep-seated abscesses. To link these progressions of disease in the 16th Century must have required a remarkable patience in observation and the brilliant discrimination of a host of other ailments themselves without any known cause or categorization.[9] Perhaps it is fitting that the primary stage of Syphilis is one of genital ulceration presenting at the seat of its acquisition and its hallmark is the soft indolent ulcer which became known as the *chancre*.[10] Although there are other sexually transmitted diseases which mimic this small ulcer, the typical *chancre* is usually quite visible, isolated and painless without any itch or irritation. It is so distinctive as to be punched out and clean with a thin exudative fluid often leaking from its centre.[11]

The danger of the chancre not being readily visible in women (the loosest of whom were considered the real Renaissance peril in the spread of Syphilis) could not have been more starkly represented by the German satirist Ulrich von Hutten when

---

[8] Even Lord Randolph's pre-morbid character which the Times described as "Gallic" hinted at the intrinsic nature of the disease. *The Times*, 25th Jan, 1895: pp. 5–6.

[9] de Vigo recorded the 'natural history' of the disease in his *Surgical Practice* of 1514 (*Practica capiosa in arte chirurgica Roma*).

[10] The word *chancre* meaning 'little ulcer' comes from the Old French and from the dominant Northwestern dialect, the *langues d'oils*, which was in vernacular use between the 9th and the 14th Centuries. The chancre was the dominant defining feature of early (and potentially treatable) Syphilis in the early 20th Century. When the Irish author James Joyce (1882–1941) contracted venereal disease his friend Oliver St. John Gogarty (1878–1957) revelled in the delight of Joyce's chancre. In a message Gogarty sent to Joyce's treating doctor as a referral Gogarty wrote *"Mr Joyce is the name of the tissues surrounding the infected part"*. [See Hayden. *Ibid.* pp 239,240. Cornell University Olin Library Joyce Collection Mss]. After his venereal experience perhaps it was too much for Joyce who dropped out of medical school. Gogarty went on to become an ear, nose and throat specialist.

[11] The chancre is usually 0.5–3 cm in size and painless, but many are painful (most likely from secondary infection) and about 10% occur in sites away from the genitals, mostly the mouth, lips or fingers. In those who have Syphilis as well as HIV, chancres may be multiple. Other ulcers which can mimic Syphilis are beyond the scope of this book designed for the public but include a condition called chancroid (due to a bacillus *Hemophilus ducreyii*), genital herpes, granuloma inguinale and lymphogranuloma venereum (both more commonly African diseases). In diagnosis of the likely sites of a chancre, the sexual ingenuity of prostitutes (who most frequently spread the disease in 17th–19th C Europe), could not be underestimated. According to Dr. J Venot of Bordeaux (reporting in the *Congrès scientifique de France* in Marseille in 1846) *"vaginal coitus is almost an exception for them; the visiting doctor* [needs] *to examine the mouth, the anus, the armpits,* etc. *as well as the vulvo-uterine passage."* Quoted in C. Quétel. *Ibid:* p. 212.

lamenting in 1519 on how he had caught the disease.[12] *"There persist within the private parts of women"* he wrote *"lesions which remain remarkably virulent for a long time....they are potentially dangerous because they are less evident to the eye......the condition* [is] *so pernicious for these lesions make it impossible to avoid the sickness because the bodies of women of this sort are sometimes so badly infected."* He had read similar reports by the physician Niccolo Leoniceno (1428–1524) written a quarter of a century before of pustules landing *"upon the privy parts"*[13] and frank description by von Hutten of his own festering genital cankers and the suffering he had endured had even led his friends to advise him towards suicide.[14]

Von Hutten no doubt had also heard of or read the pamphlet which had appeared in 1496 written by a young student of Augsberg, Joseph Grunpeck (1473–1532) suffering from Syphilis.[15] It had been written as text around two popular woodcut prints by Sebastian Brandt (1457–1521) borrowing from Brandt's original poem on the disease. In one, Brandt, who had already acquired great fame for his woodcut the 1494 *"Ship of Fools"* (*Das Narrenschiff*) places the Virgin Mary centre stage with penitent knights on her right bathed in pure light and on her left, the young Jesus discharges barbed shafts upon the afflicted clearly covered in pustules.[16] Although Grunpeck used this narrative more to advance his theory of the astrological origins of pestilence in the second woodcut (and perhaps to ingratiate himself with the Papacy), the visual impressions of the ravages of the disease and its inherent hopelessness left an indelible mark upon anyone who saw it. Grunpeck leaves no doubt concerning its stain on the genitals. "[It] *loosed its first arrow into my Priapic glans"* he wrote *"which on account of the wound became so swollen, that both hands could scarcely encircle it"*.[17]

---

[12] Ulrich von Hutten. *De guiaci medicina et morbo gallico.* Mainz 1519.

[13] Niccolo Leoniceno. *De Morbo Gallico.* Milan Venice 1497.

[14] See Claude Quétel. *History of Syphilis.* Johns Hopkins University Press Baltimore 1990: p29. Quétel's book was originally published under the title: *Le Mal de Naples* in 1986.

[15] *A treatise on the pustular epidemic Scorre or the French sickness, containing details of its origin and of the remedies for it composed by the venerable Master Josephus Grunpeck of Burckhausen following certain poems by Sebastian Brant, professor of civil and canon law. (Tractatus de pestilentiali Scorre Sive Mala de Franzos. Originem Remediaque ejusdem continens copilatus a vene rabili viro Magistro Joseph Grunpeck de Burckausen sub carmina quedam Sebastiani Brant utriusque juris professoris,* 1496).

[16] It is unclear whether the barbs in the image are causing the disease or about to cure it. The knights in the picture are headed by Emperor Maximilian I and the banner they carry bears the shield of the Hapsburg eagle, his family crest. In a later image, the barbs are replaced by rays of Divine light protecting the small clustered group of penitent sinners and the pockmarked unrepentant knight covered in sores lies in the centre of the picture below and left to die.

[17] See *Libellus Josephi Grunpeckii de mentalagra alias morbo gallico. 1503.* Although not previously suggested, (since Syphilis is not usually associated with gross oedema of the genitals), it is not inconceivable that Grunpeck may have been suffering from elephantiasis, a parasitic worm infestation that invades the body's lymphatic system and which can cause grotesque enlargement of the penis and scrotum.

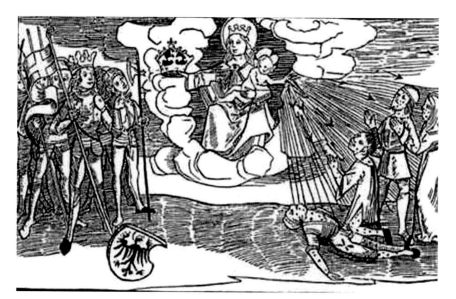

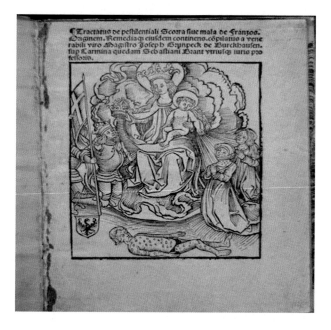

Joseph Grunpeck, Tractatus de pestilentiali Scorra sive mala de Franzos Wellcome Collection

So too did Pope Alexander VI's personal physician Pedro Pintor (1423–1503) concentrate in graphic detail his preoccupation with its beginnings in the male and female genitalia.[18] Offers of hope for cure were limited but there were always handy post-coital recommendations. Anoint the genitals with white wine but make sure to pad them dry only with towels and sheets that had never had contact with prostitutes. Rub them vigorously with the shavings of the Guiacum West Indian wood adding flakes of copper, gentian root and the grains of a charred stag's horn. For some, sever a live pigeon or a frog in twain and place the penis inside the warm bloody flesh so that its heat would draw out the poison from the inflamed member[19] or gently cover the offending chancre (once it had formed) with a spider's web.[20] The fear of God would be instilled by Johannes Benedictus morbidly obsessed with the genitals and recounting one patient of his from Venice whose penis and testicles had actually fallen off![21] The message through shock and awe was reverential; always lead a physically clean life and mental and spiritual cleanliness will follow (*mens sana in sano corpore*).[22]

Valencia's physician to the Borgia family, Gaspar Torella (1452–1520) although also writing about the gross effects on the genitalia reminded that there were other modes of intimate contact capable of spreading the disease and he was the first to point out its passage from a suckling breast to a baby's mouth.[23] But these were not sober remarks. They warned of the appalling risks to whole families of unfettered contagion and of the need for constant penitence even if the most vigilant were powerless to defend one another. In 1551, the Jewish Portuguese physician João Rodrigues de Castelo Branco, (1511–1568) better known as Amatus Lusitanus published amongst his case histories the tragedy of one family.[24] The patriarch confident that his brush with Syphilis had been long cured, unwittingly infected his wife and through the resultant pregnancy, the newborn child. From there the mother, too ill to nourish her own, handed the child over to a wet nurse who herself along with the nurse's husband became infected within the month and from there

---

[18] Petrus Pintor. *Agregator sententiarum doctorum omnium de p[reservatione et curatione pestilentiae.* Rome 1499 as *"in proeputio capitis virgae et in vulva mulierum".* Also *De morbo foedo et occulto (morbo gallico)* Rome 1500.

[19] Gruner. C-G. *Aphrodisiacus, sive de lue venereal* Jena 1789. Quoted from Aloysuis Luisinius (2 vols) 1728. Quoted in C. Quétel *Ibid* pp. 23, 282.

[20] Many like the French syphilologist Philppe Ricord (1800–1899) believed that radical excision of genital chancres would prevent the disease from becoming systemic. Coitus interruptus was widely advocated where it was traditionally contested that only an erect 'member' could have sufficient strength to ward off Syphilis (which was thought to only enter the flaccid penis).

[21] Johannis Benedicti. *De Morbo gallico libellus* 1508. See Quétel. *Ibid* 26, 282.

[22] *Transl. Lt.* A healthy mind and a healthy body.

[23] Gasparis Torellae. *Dialous de dolore, cum tractatu de ulceribus in pudendagra evenire, solitis* Rome 1500.

[24] Some regard Lusitanus as the one who really discovered the nature of the circulation of the blood before its official discoverer, William Harvey. Lusitanus published this sad story in his *De Gallica scabie. (L. Torrentino 1551)* Vol 1: p. 560. The tragic story of this family is quoted in Sir Vivian Nutton's *The Reception of Fracastoro's Theory of Contagion: The Seed that Fell Among the Thorns? Osiris* Vol 6 Renaissance Medical Learning: Evolution of a Tradition 1990: pp. 196–234, 226.

two more children she was nursing and both of their mothers as well. The first newborn and the index father who had started this small catastrophe soon died by which time the insidious disease had claimed nine new victims.

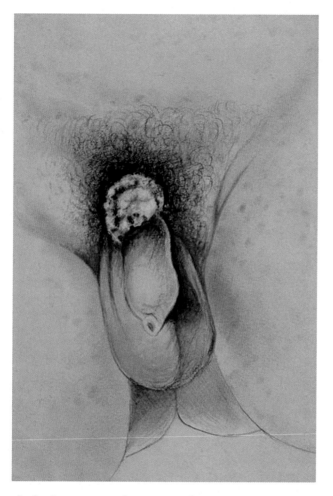

A diseased penis showing symptoms of gangrenous chancre of the pubis. Christopher D'Alton, 1866. (Watercolour with chalk, courtesy Wellcome Collection)

In most, the small quasi-innocent chancre heals although it will often leave a legacy of inflamed lymph nodes in the groin. The *buba* (as it was called) so formed, raised in some the spectre of the Black Death which had ravaged Europe some 200 years before and which had devastated its populations.[25] In the lyrical nature of

---

[25] The European Black Death raged roughly from 1346–1353 killing between 75–200 million people (between 30–60% Europe's population).

the Irish surgeon-poet Oliver St. John Gogarty (1878–1957) the central nature of the chancre was integral to diagnosis when he penned a verse after examining his friend James Joyce:

In the house where whores are dwelling

Unless it is wrapped in a glove,

A little Hunterian swelling

Poxes the part that they love.[26]

Those now entering this second stage of Syphilis became highly contagious but before its appearance they were lulled into a false sense of security with one-third even forgetting the insignificance of its preceding primary chancre. Forgotten or no, after between 4 and 10 weeks they would develop a widespread rash usually upon the torso which snaked its way onto the palms and the soles of the feet and they would become troubled with serpentine ulcers of the mouth and the tongue. At this stage, Syphilis through its distinctly cutaneous manifestations, becomes a visible disorder in a way exemplified by the skin changes of Kaposi's tumours which proved a feature of those afflicted with HIV-AIDS. In this cutaneous form it historically became a disease within the perview of the dermatologists.[27]

The skin is covered with soft fleshy papules and marks which in the rich tradition of medical description have been ascribed the qualities of food. They appear like 'raw ham' (to some) with pallid, protuberant almost elephantine excrescences that teem with microorganisms and that are hothouses of contagion.[28] In some, another almost Godly stain is a sudden moth-eaten loss of scalp hair that styles itself to the penitential tonsures of monks shaving the top of their heads in religious devotion. The mark is prominently seen in a man with his back to us in Luca Giordano's (1634–1705) 1664 painting, the *Allegory of Syphilis*. In its secondary guise, Grunpeck became *"covered from the head ....with a rough scabies ...which spares no part of the face* ...[It had become] *so filthy and repugnant,"* he wrote, that those who suffer from it could only hope for death. The *syphilides* of the skin (as they became known) marked those so afflicted like lepers and often sufferers from

---

[26] Oliver St. John Gogarty. See Hayden. *Ibid.* p. 345. Cornell University Olin Library Joyce Collection No. 31. p. 536.

[27] The dominance of the widespread rash in the secondary stage as a clinical syndrome in its own right was the reason for the historical establishment of clinics of DermatoVenereology; a marriage reflected in the specialty's journals like the *AMA Archives of Dermatology and Syphilology* which only dropped the '*and Syphilology*' title in the 1950s.

[28] Much pathology in medicine has been likened historically to foods e.g. the anchovy paste abscess of the liver in amoebic dysentery, the watermelon stomach of chronic hypertrophic gastritis, the cauliflower ear or the chocolate ovarian cyst of endometriosis. The large white protuberances are called *condylomata lata* distinguishing them from the viral *condylomata accuminata*, the result of viral infection (genital warts) which can of course coexist with Syphilis.

both complaints were hospitalized together almost as if the shame and disfigurement for both diseases was regarded with some equivalency.[29]

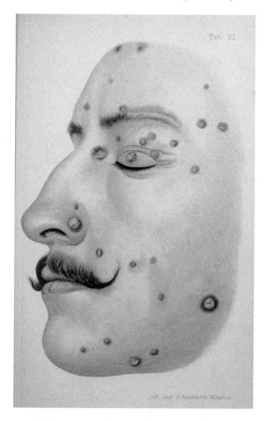

Small Pustules on the face' From 'Atlas of syphilis and the venereal diseases, including a brief treatise on the pathology and treatment' by Prof. Dr. Franz Mracek, Lemuel Bolton Bangs. 1898. Philadelphia WB Saunders. Courtesy Wellcome Collection. Attribution 4.0 International (CC BY 4.0)

---

[29] Those prostitutes with Syphilis who were so marked by the syphilide skin lesions were forcibly incarcerated in Saint-Lazare located in the 10th Arrondissement in Paris. Saint-Lazare began as a leper colony in the 12th Century founded by Louis VII and was the pilgrimage point of St. Vincent de Paul. It was converted in 1794 into a prison designed initially to house the enemies of the French Revolution and was used as an antechamber for the guillotine during the Reign of Terror. It then became a women's prison by decree of the Convention Nationale at one time incarcerating the German double agent Mata Hari. In 1835 a special infirmary wing (the *blanchisserie*) was established to care for 360 women with Syphilis. Saint-Lazare became notorious and was eventually closed in 1940 being described by the Algerian novelist Victor Margueritte (1866–1942) as *"a leprosy in the heart of Paris"*. [See Preface by V Margueritte to Jeanne-Henriette Humbert-Riaudin's *Le pourrissoir, Saint-Lazare: Choses Vues, entendues et vécues*. Paris Editions, Prima 1932]. In the words of the French magistrate Adolphe Guillot (1836–1906) *"Pour une femme, il vaut mieux mourir que d'entrer à Saint Lazare"* (*For a woman, it is better to die than to go to Saint Lazare"*) [See A. Guillot. *Des Principes du nouveau Code d'Instruction Criminelles* Paris L. Laros et Force, 1884: p.187].

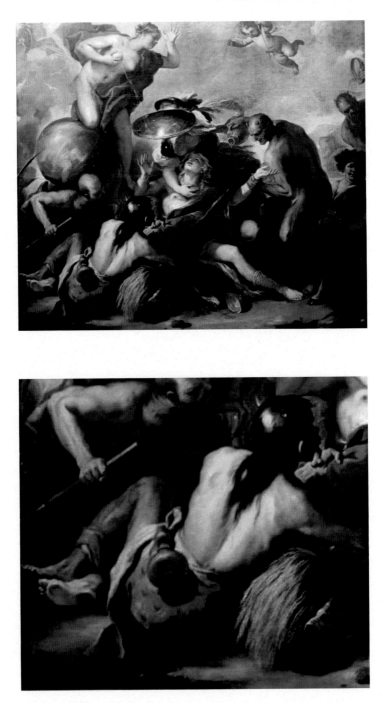

Luca Giordano. Oil on cavas. Städel Museum, Frankfurt am Main. (plus close-up of the patchy bald spot induced during the secondary stage of Syphilis)

Symptoms now assuaged, it becomes *latent* (so-called) where there is in the blood (as we shall see later) some immunological memory of disease but nothing else to signify the presence of any illness. The organism remains but out of view (and of mind) waiting to return under the cover of some new bodily stress. It bides its time so to speak until in some other state its host is weakened, susceptible and less alert. And memory such as it is, showing a semblance of recognition to the syphilitic proteins that is measurable as antibodies in the blood, steadfastly refuses to fight or to call to arms the myriad of cells which might eradicate a new syphilitic surge. It displays an immunological impotence that leads in some after 10 or even 20 years to its so-called *tertiary* stage.

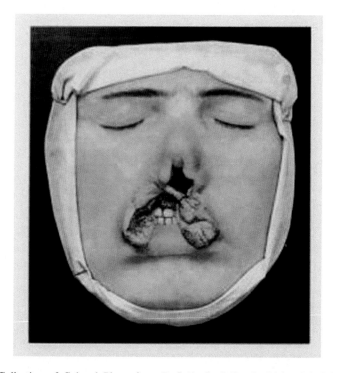

From "A Collection of Colored Plates from Prof. Bockenheimer's "Atlas der Chirurgischen Hautkrankheiten" Illustrating Interesting Surgical Conditions". New York: Rebman, (1913). Courtesy Wellcome Collection. Attribution 4.0 International (CC BY 4.0)

Now it is this stage that is of greatest clinical interest as it leads to the most exotic and notorious of presentations. In some it manifests as discrete abscesses in remote bodily locations and in others these infections lead to the most visible destructiveness. Alessandro Benedictus, a physician observing the retreat of Charles VIII's Italian expedition as it succumbed to the French at the battle of Fornovo on 5th July 1495, wrote that he saw its sufferers who had "*lost their eyes, their hands, their noses and their feet*"[30] and it is the disintegration of the integrity of the face that for some (particularly in Eastern Europe) is an enduring and entirely representative image of this disease. It had become more than a disease, acquiring the reputation of having an appetite, eating its way through the soft tissues as reprisal for past lascivious indiscretions. In this tertiary guise, Syphilis is characterized by a hard collection of viscid pus forming in the deepest locations which gradually liquefies into a firm rubbery inflammatory ball that has acquired the name *gumma* as a sign of its consistency. When I was a medical student in Melbourne in the 1970's, our anatomy and pathology museums were filled to the brim with the *gummata* of the heart, the kidneys, the liver, skull and brain and we were expected to discuss the minutest aspect of their appearance and of their unique microscopy. Back then, Syphilis was in the differential diagnosis of virtually any mass presenting anywhere in the body.[31]

Perhaps the most idiosyncratic of presentations is that where Syphilis attacks the brain substance itself or the spinal cord and its coverings and to which the label neurosyphilis can rightfully be used. Neurosyphilis is, however, not just one disease but a multiplicity of complaints, some of which confine their attacks to the meningeal coverings of the brain as a chronic meningitis, whilst others land as gummata into the central brain substance (its parenchyma so called) distorting neural fibres as they send their lines of communication between the cerebral hemispheres or out into the limbs. Not content with these destructive means, the syphilitic microorganism uniquely lands in the channels of the small microvasculature and obliterates the tiniest arteriolar blood supply to the brain substance.[32] In one other specific variant, it selectively injures the dorsal spinal column integrally concerned with providing the information to the brain about where each limb is in space and leading to a progressive (and frequently exquisitely painful) paralysis called *Tabes dorsalis*.[33] Each mode of attack creates its own unique clinical condition. In some there will be a constant headache of meningeal irritation with

---

[30] Alexandrii Benedicti *Veronensis physici historiae corporis humani* 1497. Also described by Benedetti in his *Diaria de Bello Carolino* 1495 (Available 1967 *transl. Dorothy M. Schullian, New York)*. Quoted in Quétel C. *Ibid* p10. The physician and poet John Armstrong (1709–1779) in his *Oeconomy of Love* (1736) had specifically warned against congress with prostitutes because of the risk of collapse of the nose. [See *English Poetry. Fulltext dbase. Pt II. 1600–1800.* Cambridge Engl, Alexandria Va. Chadwick-Healy 1994].

[31] The second way that tertiary Syphilis presents is as cardiovascular disease, particularly attacking the origins of the aorta as it leaves the aortic valve, causing a large thoracic aortic enlargement (an aneurysm). In the pre-Penicillin era, it was thought that cardiovascular Syphilis accounted for about 10% of all clinical cardiovascular disease and was present at autopsy in up to half of the known cases of Syphilis. Cardiovascular Syphilis is now exceptionally rare in the developed world.

[32] This particular presentation is rather unique to Syphilis resulting in a chronic inflammatory change in the small blood vessels (particularly those which provide a blood supply to small nerves). The inner layers of the vessels become heaped up and obliterated in an inflammatory response which pathologists call *endarteritis obliterans*. This results in rapid occlusion of the peripheral blood vessels.

[33] The swiftness and suddenness of painful exacerbations of Tabes are referred to clinically as tabetic crises.

destruction of the auditory nerve leading to intractable ringing in the ears (a tinnitus) and to deafness. In another an epileptic reactivity to an enlarging gumma confuses it with almost any brain tumour. Still another closing off the critical blood supply to oxygen-starved neurologic tracts would mimic a garden variety stroke. Each of these will vie with other far more common conditions as the cause of neurologic impairment with some grandiloquently claiming that Beethoven's and the Czech composer Smetana's deafness or Schumann's trials with tinnitus were syphilitic in their origins.[34]

By 1913, the Japanese-American researcher Hideyo Noguchi (1876–1928) had discovered the syphilitic bacterium lurking in the brains of those who had died with neurosyphilis. But in an age where there was no discrete means of diagnosis (and still today where there are no features on a CAT or MRI brain scan which are pathognomonic of Syphilis), some had warned of its overdiagnosis.[35] After this, almost every strange presentation confined to the asylums across Europe was presumptively labelled as syphilitic. Between 1850 and 1940 in the Edinburgh central district alone, the Lothian Health Board reported that 20% of patients hospitalized in the city's asylums had a diagnosis of neurosyphilis and that once its presence had been confirmed that it proved universally fatal.[36] But patients were lumped together in many institutions under the rubric of 'paralytic dementia' including those suffering the chronic effects of alcoholism, the delayed consequences of head trauma and the psychological sequel of 'shellshock' induced by the horrors of World War 1. Many would ultimately claim that up to one-third of those

---

[34] The composer Bedrich Smetana (1824–1884) ended his days in the Katericky Lunatic Asylum in Prague wracked with depression, insomnia and a constant ringing in his ears. Exhumation of his remains was inconclusive as to whether the cause of his death was neurosyphilis.

[35] Dr William Gowers (1845–1915) a prominent British neurologist complained of the over-diagnosis of neurosyphilis in asylums in his Lettsomian Lecture "*Syphilis and the Nervous System*" delivered to the Medical Society of London in 1889. It has since been argued in neurologic textbooks that the changing demography of modern neurologic illness recalls rare diseases of the past but no longer reflects such a legacy. As quoted by Sir Francis MR Walshe (1885–1973) the Consultant neurologist to the British Forces during World War 1, "*The belief that syphilis is the commonest single cause of organic nervous disease dies hard. It is a legacy from the textbooks of the end of the last century, in virtue of which syphilis of the nervous system occupies the place of honor, as though by merit raised to that bad eminence, in most accounts of disease of the nervous system.*" [See Sir Francis MR Walshe. *Diseases of the Nervous System*. London & Baltimore Williams & Wilkins 6th Edn 1949; p. 163]. Charles Mauriac (1832–1905) principal physician at the Hôpital du Midi claimed that "*over eager pathologists ....[have] dreamed up and taken to the extreme the conquest of the brain by syphilis*" In Charles Mauriac. *Nouvelles leçons sur les maladies vénériennes. Syphilis tertiaire*. Paris 1889 Quoted in Quetel. *Ibid* p. 165.

[36] Lothian Health Services Archives Edinburgh University Library 1908: Report Thomas Clouston LHB7/14/8:p9 and Royal Edinburgh Asylum (REA) Annual Reports 1840 and 1908. LHB 7/7/6–12. By the end of the First World War, the diagnosis rivalled that of cancer with George Robertson the REA superintendent between 1908–1932 declaring in the Morison lecture on mental health in the UK in 1913 that GPI had a 50% mortality at one year after diagnosis rising to 75% by 2 years and 90% at 3 years. Along with a falling birth rate after the Great War and the loss of young men in combat, neurosyphilis was considered the principal killer of Britain's younger male working class. [See Robertson G. *The Morison lectures* 1913. In *Journal of Mental Science* 1913: pp. 185–221].

neurosyphilitics languishing in Europe's asylums by the early 20th Century had actually been misdiagnosed.

In amongst all this misery, however, lay an almost unique presentation of neurosyphilis which became a hallmark of the disease. It coupled an irregularity of speech with tremulous incoordination and in many a sort of 'mental extinction' linked to a paralysis that gained it the evocative name *General Paresis of the Insane* (or simply *GPI*). The cognitive dissonance was remarkable combining wild delusions of grandeur with a rambling tepid enfeeblement. Nothing on earth presented quite like it where there was the promise of greatness manacled to one far too disinterested and meek to ever sally forth in any proposed achievement.[37] It represents a unique inability by the sufferer to grasp the seriousness of their complaint even on the brink of death. A man or woman who promises the world to all their imbecilic companion inmates in proximity and someone so magnanimous to accede to the simplest request and to debase themselves with the slightest intonation, climbing down from what they perceive as the loftiest pedestal to obligingly perform the most menial of tasks. London's Wellcome Institute Fellow in the history of medicine, Gayle Davis would have us believe that they approach life blissfully unaware of impending death and unprepared like one who still had the cognitive understanding of any terminal illness. And in their happy ignorance, they construct no impenetrable shell like that which forms a protective hollow and unresponsive forcefield around someone with advanced dementia. In the absence of any definitive test, the diagnosis of GPI was the only one of its type in the asylum amongst all the psychiatric mélange, only ever made in retrospect (and entirely by exclusion) with postmortem confirmation of the congested thickened meninges. By definition, those who had survived or whose lunacy had even improved under watchful eyes simply could not have had the disease.[38]

---

[37] Presentations of GPI were notably eclectic. Dr. Davis describes cases characterized by extraordinary grandiosities, with one example claiming to have married hundreds of women, along with the usual mad ones with a God complex. [See G. Davis. *The most deadly disease of asylumdom: General paralysis of the insane and Scottish psychiatry, c. 1840–1940. Journal of the Royal College of Physicians of Edinburgh.* 2012; 42: pp. 266–273].

[38] The sheer prevalence of GPI cases in asylums across Great Britain prompted the psychiatrist Sir James Crichton-Browne (1840–1938) to use photographs of his patients as part of their medical record. His father Dr William AF Browne (1805–1885) who established and reformed some of Britain's asylums and who was a seminal influence on the young Charles Darwin (1809–1882), was also an active member of the Edinburgh Phrenological Society using cranial measurements to establish personality and character traits. The phrenological background and the family connection with Darwin stimulated a long period of correspondence between James and Darwin with Crichton-Browne developing an atlas of neuropsychiatric photographs and the influential monograph the *West Riding Lunatic Asylum Medical Reports* between 1869 and 1975 at Wakefield. Many of the photographs became iconic impressions of Victorian madness and this approach might have been stimulated by Darwin sending Crighton-Browne a copy of Duchenne de Boulogne's (1806–1875) *Mechanism of Human Facial Expression* which contained pioneering photographs of electrical stimulation of facial twitch muscles in living patients. Darwin ultimately used a single photograph sent to him by Crichton-Browne for his 1872 book *The Expression of the Emotions in Man and Animals.*

The 19th Century saw the paired rise of the specialties of neurology and psychiatry, both driven forwards by their champions Emil Kraepelin, (1856–1926) Aloysius Alzheimer (1864–1915) and Jean-Martin Charcot (1825–1893). In Munich, Kraepelin had established his Institute for Psychiatric Research and was instrumental in decriminalizing insanity in Germany moving many of the mentally ill from the prisons to asylums. Charcot in his Salpêtrière School of Hypnosis had established the very architecture of the field of neurology with his public demonstrations of the visible effects of hysteria and his technique of open display of a patient's symptoms and signs became the method of medical training amongst many specialties. It had converted clinical medicine into a regulated science of exposure with the aim of inducing a pattern recognition of signs and an emulation of their eliciting techniques. But in so doing, it had turned diseases like GPI into vignettes of showy exposition that could rival the public lust for any local freak show. The 1820s saw the young alienist[39] Antoine-Laurent Bayle (1799–1858) first separating out an illness which became GPI from all the other neurological dross pervading the streets of Paris and by 1822 he had linked the clinical mix of madness with ambitious mania and progressive generalized paralysis with a chronic inflammatory arachnoiditis in the brains of those who had died from Syphilis.[40]

Of all the French clinicians, Philippe Ricord (1800–1889) was probably the first to separate the main venereal diseases (gonorrhoea and syphilis) dispelling the dogma of the British surgeon John Hunter (1728–1793) that they were one and the same disorder and Ricord was the first to consider Syphilis in its protean stages creating in effect, some new boundaries for the disease.[41] Ricord's protégé Jean Alfred Fournier (1832–1914) who started life as a dermatologist, became the father of venereology establishing it as a distinct specialty and beginning a dedicated clinic at the Lourcine Hospital in 1876. Fournier was the first syphilologist to link prior syphilitic infection with the creeping locomotor ataxia that filled the medical wards. He was successful in making the connection by using the available statistics and merely correlating the number of neurological cases with a known previous bout of Syphilis.[42] Although most believe that he also linked GPI to Syphilis, his statistics in this area were far less robust and at first even he was reluctant to make that connection.[43]

---

[39] An archaic term for psychiatrist.

[40] A-L-J Bayle, *Récherches sur l'arachnite chroni gue, Ia gastrite et Ia gastro-enterite chroni gues, et Ia goutte, considérée conime causes de l'aliénation mentale* (Paris: Didot le Jeune, 1822), *transl* by M Moore and H C Solomon.

[41] [See P Ricord, *Traité Pratique des Maladies Vénériennes, ou Récherches critiques et experimentales sur l'inoculation appliqué a l'étude de ses maladies …* (Paris: J Rouvier et E Le Bouvier, 1838].

[42] JA Fournier. *De L'ataxie locomotrice d'origine syphilitigue* (1876).

[43] JA Fournier. *La Syphilis du Cerveau* 1879. Both Friedrich von Esmarch (1823–1908) and Peter Willers Jessen, (1793–1875) two Scandinavian alienists had suggested a link between GPI and Syphilis as early as 1857 (well before Fournier) but neither had been recognized in the Syphilis literature.

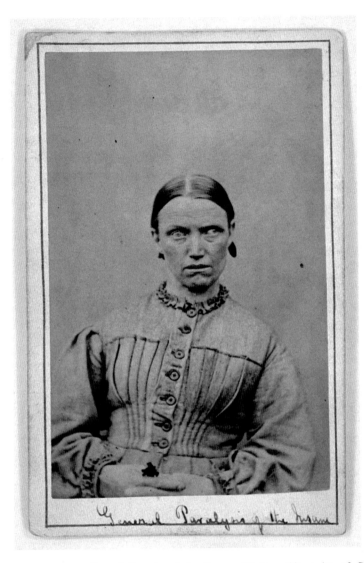

Woman suffering from General Paresis of the Insane. Photographic series of Sir James Crichton-Browne. Ca 1869. [The patient was Elizabeth Hardcastle, a patient at the West Riding Lunatic Asylum, Wakefield Yorkshire]. (Courtesy of the Wellcome Library London). Courtesy Wellcome Collection. Attribution 4.0 International (CC BY 4.0)

One final horrendous scourge is congenital syphilis, a disease so pervasive that it had established its own clinical laws of behaviour.[44] In the 1930s it was so prevalent that the Hospital for Sick Children in Great Ormond Street held the unique distinction of being the only children's hospital in London which was part of the Venereal Diseases Scheme of the London City Council. Children afflicted typically presented with a classical coryza 'the snuffles' as it was benignly called that left them with a continuous runny nose, breathing difficulties and inflamed eyes. Their bones were the seat of chronic persistent inflammation that systematically destroyed the growth plate of almost any bone and joint. Open their mouths and the legacy was obvious. Their central incisor teeth were spaced far apart and cut in their centres with thick crude notches and the molars (when visible) were dumb-bell shaped and inflamed.[45] According to the Belfast alienist Samuel AK Strahan, (1853–1902) the children each looked like sick little old men and were in stark contrast to their healthy peers. *"All syphilitic children are ill-developed, miserable, puny things"*, he wrote in his 1892 book on *The Diseases of Marriage.* " *Their little faces are withered, pale, and pinched; their noses become flat, their heads are large ... their cheeks seared with the scars of old sores; and over all there is a strange uncanny look of age and suffering which is repulsive, and strangely at variance with the cherub-like features and innocence of the healthy infant".*[46] But many of these florid descriptions had confused the deformed bony

---

[44] There was much confusion as to whether the father or the mother was the main infective risk to the infant. Heredo-familial Syphilis was governed (some said) by Kassowitz's Law which suggested that in an untreated woman the organism responsible became progressively more attenuated. In this Law she was expected to first experience a period of sterility, followed by several spontaneous abortions and miscarriages, then a stillbirth or two and finally the birth of a child sick with congenital disease. Similarly Diday's Law of Decrease suggested that the disease would in some attenuate where premature stillbirths would be followed by full-term stillbirths and ultimately the birth of a normal live infant. Some attested to Colles' Law (so named by Hutchinson after Abraham Colles an 18th Century Dublin physician) which stated that the mother of a newborn syphilitic infant infected by the father would be immune to infection herself. It is also expressed as the fact that syphilitic infants could not infect their birth mother but could infect a healthy wet nurse. The real meaning, however, was that the mother was already infected. Profeta's Law articulated in 1865 suggested that an apparently healthy baby born of a syphilitic mother cannot be infected by her.

[45] So-called Hutchinson's incisors and Moon's mulberry molars.

[46] Strahan S.A.K. *Marriage and Disease: A Study of Heredity and the More Important Family Degenerations* (London: Kegan Paul, Trench, Tribner & Co, 1892); pp. 143, 152. The Glasgow obstetrician John Burns also wrote in 1811 *"sometimes it has at the time of birth or soon afterwards acquired a wrinkled countenance having the appearance of old age in miniature, so very remarkably, that no one who has ever seen such a child can possibly forget the look of the petit vieillard".* [See J Burns. *The Principles of Midwifery; Including the Diseases in Women and Children.* 2nd Edn. London Longman and Hurst, Rees, Orme and Browne. 1811: pp. 485–9]. Jean Astruc put it more bluntly in his *Treatise of the Venereal Diseases* writing that the infants are *"squalid, erysipelatous, half-rotten, ulcerated Foetus's....strumous, rickety, gibbous, hectical, lean...and if they live, are short, broken-backed, large headed, crooked, bandy-legged, variously distorted and thick jointed."* From *A Treatise on the Venereal Diseases in Six Books Containing an Account of the Origins, Propagation and Contagion of this Distemper. Transl* William Barrowby MD 1737. Reprint New York Da Capo Press 1972; pp. 52, 56.

symptomatology with the Vitamin D deficiency rickets so pervasive amongst malnourished children. Rickets too had shown similar cranial and facial deformities as Syphilis with the same sort of sloping brow, the turret-shaped head and the sunken saddle-like nose.

Congenital Syphilis had provoked the most vociferous debates principally concerning how it was transmitted to the child. Was it in the sperm of the father or did the child contract the disease passing through an infected womb?[47] Some no doubt were infected under the practice of farming children out to professional wet nurses. The fear from congenital Syphilis which seemed to reach its height in France was that these syphilitic infants would grow up into contaminating adults; men and women capable of tainting an entire population. The peril then would be at one and the same time, both personal and collective and it would even threaten to derail the path of human progress only just outlined by the greatest philosophical minds of the Enlightenment.[48] It had led to the confusion between the 'hereditaries' (contracted in utero) and the 'congenitals' (contracted from an infected wet nurse) that so terrified not only the doctors but also the masses in general. Of course they were all congenital cases.[49] It had taken on a decidedly ominous fear during France's Ancien régime and had latched itself to a whole class of miscreants who one imagined were roaming the streets and carelessly impregnating unsuspecting women with their syphilitic seed. This then was the feared band of society's 'hérédos'. As if to reflect the crisis, the literature abounded with its own cases even when the physicians had no clue either how it had arrived or how to contain it. Daniel Defoe (1660–1731) in homage to its familial legacy had written of its risk to the "*life blood of posterity*" in the bawdy tale of Moll Flanders[50] and Jonathan Swift (1667–1745) had scathed afterwards on the limits to any likely issue that Syphilis would impose upon a family. The progeny of the idle nobility would soon enough "*contract odious diseases among lewd females*" Swift prophesied ... "*the*

---

[47] Much of the confusion during the 18th and 19th Centuries lay in poor diagnosis and distinction from gonorrhoea where babies presenting with a running ophthalmitis had acquired it from passage through the maternal genital tract infected with gonorrhoea.

[48] See Barbara J. Dunlap. Ch 7. *The problem of syphilitic children in Eighteenth Century France and England*. In *The Secret Malady. Venereal Disease in Eighteenth Century Britain and France*. Linda E. Merians (Ed) University Press of Kentucky 1996 pp 114–127.

[49] See David Nunes Nabarro. *Congenital Syphilis*, London E. Arnold 1934.

[50] Daniel Defoe. *Fortunes and Misfortunes of the Famous Moll Flanders*. 1722. Ed GA Starr London Oxford University Press 1971; p. 227.

productions of [their] *Marriages are generally scrophulous, rickety or deformed children; by which means the family seldom continues above three generations*".[51]

By July 1780, its high prevalence had provoked Jean Lenoir, (1732–1807) the Lieutenant Général de Police in Paris to open a hospice totally dedicated to the care of the venereal infant and he saved the precious milk of those lactating women who came to the new Hôpital de Vaugirard for their daily mercurial friction rubs, ensuring its distribution to all the sick babies.[52] Under a ruling by Jules Parrot (1829–1883) in 1881, a *nouricerrie* (nourishment centre) was opened where donkey milk was brought from specially tended stables located on site at the hospital for the purpose so that clean wet nurses were not secondarily infected by the suckling children. Parrot's pavilion (as it became known) was immortalized in a painting by the Dutch artist Frédéric de Haenen (1853–1928) in 1887 who is perhaps best known for his work the *Degradation of Captain Alfred Dreyfus*.[53] The practice of providing animal milk was widespread with as far back as 1612 the *Manual of Nursing and Bringing Up of Children* by Jacques Guillemeau (1550–1613) advocating that "*if you cannot find a Nurse that will venture to give the children suck... instead thereof you shall cause it to suck a Goate*".[54]

---

[51] Jonathan Swift. *Gulliver's Travels*. 1726 a.k.a. *Travels into Several Remote Nations of the World. In Four Parts. By Lemuel Gulliver, First a Surgeon, and then a Captain of Several Ships*, 2nd Edn Ed Paul Turner Oxford Oxford University Press 1986 Ed; p. 261.aul Turner Oxford Oxford University Press 1986 Ed; p. 261.

[52] Public health was traditionally considered a police matter in 18th Century Paris as was the criminal responsibility of controlling prostitution. Remarkably, syphilitic infants who were breast fed under the scheme survived longer than those babies who did not have Syphilis but who were left languishing malnourished and denied breast milk in the foundling Bicêtre hospital across the other side of the city. The Hôpital de Vaugirard (specifically for Syphilitic children) did not remain open long and closed in 1793 with the syphilitic infants transferred to the Hôpital des Vénériens in the Couvent des Capucins. (under the auspices of the Franciscan order of Capuchin monks).

[53] de Haenen F: La nourricerie du pavillon Par- rot (oil on canvas). Paris, Musée de l'Assistance Publique.

[54] Directly putting the child to suckle onto the animal was it was believed the only way of preventing the spread of infection. See Jacques Guillemeau *The Manual of Nursing and Bringing Up of Children*. 1612 Reprint New York Da Capo Press 1972 (Ed); pp. 114–115, 119.

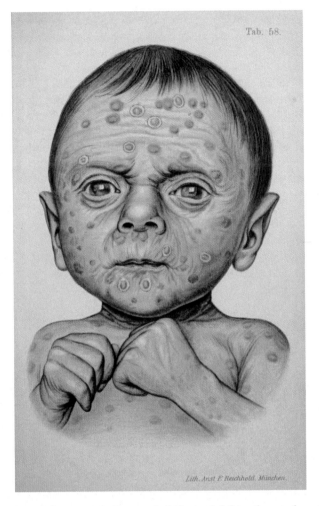

Atlas of syphilis and the venereal diseases, including a brief treatise on the pathology and treatment by Prof. Dr. Franz Mracek, 1898. [Patient S.K. at 4 weeks of age in July 1897 died of pneumonia and hepatitis, confirmed at autopsy]. Courtesy Wellcome Collection. Attribution 4.0 International (CC BY 4.0)

The side issue of the European wet nurse too (and her place in society) was something which had been very regulated by Governments as it was a National source of revenue, particularly in France where the aristocracy would employ them in-house. The middle class not to be outdone would also send their infants away to the country for feeding. On this background, the Government actually sometimes did more to facilitate than curtail the spread of disease.[55] In Paris, the Hôpital Vaugirard accepted the city's paupers and at least provided treatment for her syphilitic mothers whose milk would be able to transmit to their sickly infants some of the mercury they had been administered. Even when the majority of the children sick enough to come through its doors would die, their chances of survival were better than they might have been at any of the other Foundling hospitals across the city.

By the 1950s congenital Syphilis had become rare in most developed countries but I am ashamed to say that as a young doctor in the late 1980s working in Darwin in Australia's far north, I still saw my fair share of cases of young aboriginal babies dying from the disease with their tragic autopsies revealing the characteristically unique white solid lungs and non-functional white livers.[56] Nowadays, with maternal screening and the wide availability of Penicillin (to which the organism has not gained resistance), congenital Syphilis has become a medical curiosity in the developed world. But it is sadly showing a global resurgence with the World Health Organization reporting recently that up to half a million children will die annually from this entirely preventable disease.[57] Our own Aboriginal population in Australia has been experiencing since 2011 its highest incidence of treatable Syphilis on record which speaks volumes on health equity and access in a first world country.[58]

Syphilis had now been named even if it lingered only in the poetry of an age almost powerless to protect its citizens from contagion. Its harmful clinical expressions could be identified and its progression documented from the contaminating seats of its genital entry through a complacent dormancy and thence to a bizarre set of idiosyncratic maladies. It had spared no one, least of all the moralists who in rounding up and imprisoning their prostitutes had shifted the disease to unregistered women and girls. The 20th Century would find the microscopic culprit, develop serology that could monitor the body's immune response to disease and promulgate the antibiotic that would cast off medieval treatments and their toxicities. It would sequence the organism's genome and postulate an ancestral partnership permitting bacterium and host to coexist and it would spawn a few Nobel prizes along the way.

---

[55] [See Valerie Fildes. *Wet-nursing: a history from Antiquity to the Present*. Oxford Basil Blackwell 1988 and also George Sussman. *Selling Mother's Milk: The Wet-nursing Business in France. 1715–1914*. Urbana University of Illinois Press 1982].

[56] So-called *pneumonia alba* and *hepar alba*.

[57] Congenital Syphilis is still implicated in one-fifth of every perinatal sub-Saharan death and 1% of all paediatric admissions in Africa. This is despite the World Health Organization (WHO) launching a global initiative to eliminate the disease in 2006. This neonatal toll easily exceeds that of HIV.

[58] There are a number of medical reports on an outbreak in the northern states and territory of Australia between 2011 and 2019 which included reported congenital cases. See for example Rode NB, Ryder N and Su J-Y. An audit on the management and outcomes of infants at risk of congenital syphilis in the Top End of the Northern Territory, Australia, 2005–2013. Commun Dis Intell 2018; 42:S2209-S6051 (18): 00,018–0.

Chapter 4
In Search of the Organism and a Zauberkugeln (Magic Bullet) for Treatment[*]

What should mankind undertake when all diseases have been eradicated?
Eduard von Hartmann (1842–1906) in a letter to Emil von Behring (1854–1917)

Abstract After Paul Erich Hoffmann (1868–1959) and Fritz Richard Schaudinn (1871–1906) first saw the causative bacillus of Syphilis under the microscope in 1905, the enigmatic researcher Hideyo Noguchi (1876–1928) was able to find the organism in the brains and spinal cords of patients who had died of neurosyphilis. Since the Treponema bacterium cannot be cultured in the laboratory outside of an animal (monkeys and rabbits), a range of blood tests showing active or latent anti-Syphilis immunity (the VDRL-Wasserman test, the TPHA, TPI or FTA test) are used in diagnosis. The brief story of the development and developers of these tests is discussed. The salves for disease are considered, with mercurials taken orally or in

---

[*]*German* meaning 'Magic Bullet'. In the quest for the eradication of infectious diseases, the German researcher Paul Ehrlich (1854–1915) proposed the theory of the side-chain' where infective agents would externally expose alien receptor molecules (antigens) to which attractant molecules (antibodies) would circulate and join. His theoretical assertion was that chemically based magic bullets (*Zauberkugeln*) could be designed to lock onto the antigens of any infectious disease without inducing toxicity. He first used the term in his Harben Lectures at the Royal Institute of Public Health in London in 1908 in a lecture entitled: *Experimental Researches on Specific Therapy. On Immunity with Special Reference to the Relationship Between Distribution and Action of Antigens.* It was the first time that a specific type of 'chemotherapy' (as it became known) for the treatments of parasitic disease (and ultimately for cancer) was proposed. The 'lock-and-key' hypothesis was the forerunner of an understanding of human immunity with the concept of chemically structured 'designer' antibodies as definitive therapies. It was in Ehrlich's nature to define the defeat of disease as an intrinsically chemical phenomenon in the absence of any understanding of the genetic mutational events that occur in microorganisms to induce antibiotic resistance or in cancers to evade novel chemotherapeutic agents. The German word *Zauberkügel* has been compared by Bernhard Witkop to the word *Freikugel* (Free Ball) first used in Carl von Weber's opera *Der Freischütz* a folkloric tale of a marksmanship contest in the German woods. [See B Witkop. Paul Ehrlich and his Magic Bullets—Revisited. In Proceedings of the American Philosophical Society 1999; 143: pp. 540–557]. Ehrlich's concepts were the precursor of ideas concerning cellular receptors and he had been tossing up terminology in his mind for new structures which would attack harmful parasites but not injure the host organism. Witkop argues unconvincingly that the *Zauberkügel* would be better termed a *Zauberschrot* (magic 'buckshot').

friction rubs or as sweating vapours the mainstay for half a millennium. Given the terrible litany of side-effects (the rotting of teeth, hair loss and a shaking palsy) there were staunch anti-mercurialists promoting a range of quack therapies until Paul Ehrlich (1854–1915) hit upon his arsenical compound Salvarsan. It proved so successful in injectable form that hundreds of thousands of doses were shipped to the front-line battlefields of WW1. But following some deaths with Salvarsan and a harrowing court case brought against Ehrlich (which he won) interest in this drug fell away. For a short while the malaria therapy of Julius Wagner-Jauregg (1857–1940) became fashionable in a design to sweat the spirochaete out of the body by super-infecting patients with a malarial parasite. The discovery by Alexander Fleming (1881–1955) of Penicillin was tested in June 1943 in the VDRL research facility in Staten Island on 4 patients with early Syphilis completely eradicating their disease and causing a world sensation. As with Salvarsan, Penicillin was shipped to the European theatre of War where it showed many other valuable uses. But appearance of a wonder drug that the New York Times confidently and prematurely declared in a 1944 editorial spelled *"the end of Syphilis"* proved wildly inaccurate.

It is perhaps surprising that the organism responsible for Syphilis was only discovered a little more than one hundred years ago. This finding occurred in a world where the principal microbiological imperatives were defined more by the exotic nature of epidemics (that felled equally exotic races) than by the impression of more urgent social needs. The relatively slow, progressive acquisition of data at the start of the 20th Century concerning the Western scourge of Syphilis might be compared with the initially slow deployment of scientific resources to identify the causative organism of HIV-AIDS in the early 1980s.

Of course, finding such a small bacillus required the advent of microscopes sufficiently powerful for its detection, but Antonie van Leeuwenhoek (1632–1723) had already fashioned the delicate lenses necessary for his single-viewing instruments almost 200 years before and the machinery for the detection of the spirochaete was already there waiting.[1] Today, it seems astonishing that knowledge of small single and multicellular organisms did not translate into their implication in infective (and particularly contagious) disease for a further two centuries. But for Syphilis before the microbe was ever identified, there would be many theories concerning its genesis. Most in the 17th and 18th Centuries subscribed to a chemical thesis behind its beginnings and its spread. The physician Jean Astruc (1684–1766) chronicling the natural history of Syphilis in Montpellier was convinced of its inherently chemical nature and reactions, noting its ability to function

---

[1] Van Leeuwenhoek's earlier observations using the microscope appeared in a letter submitted to the Royal Society London on 28th April 1673 concerning the structure of moulds, parts of the anatomy of a bee and sections of a louse. The revised nature of his discovery concerning the first observation of protozoa, his 'little animals' (*kleijne diertgens*) and the bacteria 'incredibly small organisms' (*ongelooflijk kleijn*) which 'moved quickly' (*vaardige voortgang*), both of which he had observed in a single drop of rainwater, appeared in a letter to the Royal Society of London on 9th October 1676 [Mss. Royal Society London L1.22].

like a corrosive acid as it induced ulcerations, or as a blood coagulant drawing the soft tissues into hard indurated masses. For Astruc, Syphilis even demonstrated properties akin to a tissue fixative; a feature which merited it unique capabilities to move from one person to another by the most intimate contact.[2] Modernists like Leiden's Professor of Medicine Herman Boerhaave (1668–1738) had not entirely dispensed with the notion that Syphilis somehow represented a distinctly humoral imbalance although this failed as a theory to adequately describe the variant manifestations of the same disease. Nevertheless, he believed that Syphilis acted upon the bodily humors as a unique poison.[3]

It took the essayist Nicolas Andry de Bois-Regard (1658–1742) to first propose in his treatise *De la génération des vers dans les corps de l'homme* (first published in 1700) that contagions might actually be caused by what he called "worms" [4] and it is only from this point on that the Germ Theory (more commonly referred to as the Parasitic Theory) itself germinated. In a hybrid of tenets and in order to form a new so-called doctrine of sympathy, Paul-Joseph Barthez (1734–1806) Montpellier's staunch advocate of the vital principle (*le principe vitale*) which he believed animated all living things, had created a novel maxim that permitted the venereal 'virus' (whatever that may have been) to enter the body and to induce its pathology in other organs. It was only over time he felt, that the viscera would fall into a degrading syphilitic sympathy with the inflammation already commenced at the first point of entry.[5]

---

[2] This 'chemical' approach is suggested by Quétel. *Ibid* p. 78.

[3] Boerhaave was highly respected throughout Europe. Although tantalizingly close to understanding that Syphilis was due to a bacillus, he proposed that the agent of its infection somehow could penetrate the pores of the skin to produce humoral imbalance. His view formed the preface to Christian Gottfried Gruner's (1744–1815) 1728 edition of *Aphrodisiacus sive de Lue Venera*.

[4] This new theory was published in English under the title *An Account of the Breeding of Worms in Human Bodies* in 1701. A basic germ theory had also been proposed before that universally followed from the experimental work of Louis Pasteur (1822–1895) by the naturalist Francesco Redi (1626–1697). Redi was one of the first to debunk the theory that infections resulted from spontaneous generation (a so-called *abiogenesis* that life arose from non-living matter) and replace it with the genesis of disease where "*Omne vivum ex vivo*—all life derives from life"). He accomplished this through seminal work showing the transformation of maggots into flies reported in his *Esperienze Intorno alla Generazione degl'Insetti* (*Experiments on the Generation of Insects*), published in 1668. Similar work was conducted by the priest Lazzaro Spallanzani (1729–1799) whose experimentation with insects inspired Pasteur and by the French abbott Antoine Deidier (1670–1746) in his *Dissertation sur les maladies vénériennes* of 1733 who postulated that the 'venereal virus' contained small living worms which multiplied through copulation. The Germ Theory of infection was also advanced by Agostino Bassi (1773–1856) an entomologist who proposed the spread of silkworm infection by caterpillars contaminated by contagious living microorganisms in his *Del mal del segno, calcinaccio o moscardino* in 1835.

[5] Paul-Joseph Barthez. *Nouveaux elements de laa science de l'Homme*. Montpellier 1778.

The disparate theories of the generation of Syphilis were put to rest, however, with its visualization. The wriggling spiral organism responsible for Syphilis, the spirochaete, had only been definitively seen in 1905 in the material from scrapings drawn from a pustular papule taken from the vulval skin of a young prostitute by the dermatologist Paul Erich Hoffmann (1868–1959). The finding was only made (both strangely and fortuitously), when Hoffman had sent it to a local Prussian zoologist Fritz Richard Schaudinn (1871–1906), a man far more interested in the parasites of domestic poultry, ducks and owls than in any human communicable disease.[6] Originally calling the organisms *Spirochaeta* because of their spiral morphology and twisting movements, Schaudinn ultimately categorized them as within the genus *Treponema*[7] and subcategorized it as *Treponema pallidum* because of its pale appearance under the microscope. The real-time appearance of the tightly wound spiral bacterium was characteristic with its unique twisting around its long spinal axis, its hypnotic forward and backward flexing and its gymnastic lateral flicks like those of a sidewinder snake.

Even though Schaudinn and Hoffmann had rapidly demonstrated the same unique organism in many fresh syphilitic specimens, its initial appearance as the causative agent of Syphilis like so many scientific discoveries was singularly contentious. This small 'miracle' was not greeted without scientific impediment and the spread of the *T. pallidum* as the definitive cause of Syphilis was far from smooth.[8] For the scourge of the era, sufficient confusion had been created at the

---

[6] Schaudinn hit upon the idea of demonstrating the spirochaete by dark ground (or dark field) microscopy where he combined an ordinary compound microscope with a dark field condenser. The effect was to deflect most of the direct light rays away from the lens so that only peripheral angulated light was directed onto the specimen. In it, the spirochaete appeared as a tightly coiled silver thread on a completely black background. Experience of demonstrating the small organism was gained by finding its benign cousin the *Treponema microdentium* living in the mouths of healthy volunteers. Although this organism was shallower and more angulated than its 'malignant' counterpart the *Treponema pallidum* responsible for Syphilis, both treponemes looked essentially similar.

[7] The genus includes the *Borrelia* species (a group of tick-borne parasitic infections causing Lyme disease and relapsing fever) and the *Leptospirae* (responsible for the haemorrhagic kidney failure also called Weil's disease).

[8] Schaudinn and Hoffmann's work was officially overseen by one of the esteemed bacteriologists Fred Neufeld (1869–1945) who had been working with Professor Robert Koch (1843–1910). As it was, the pronouncement in favour of the *T. pallidum* as the cause of Syphilis was made in a singularly obscure journal after Neufeld (for some reason) had abandoned the research group. The false attribution of the cause to the *Cytorrhyctes* parasite was made with the comment that it was also the cause of hand-foot and mouth disease.

start of 1905 when on February 2nd the zoologist Franz Eilhard Schulze (1840–1921) had emphatically reported to the Royal Prussian Academy of Sciences that his assistant, John Siegel had definitely identified the causative agent as a small protozoon parasite the *Cytorrhyctes luis*.[9] By May 17th they were prepared to present their data to the Berlin Medical Society although there was vociferous argument between the two sides.[10] To complicate matters, the presenters at the meeting from either side were also both pupils of Schulze, both had only minimal international reputations and both were using similar samples, similarly powered microscopes and identical cell staining techniques. And to add to the confusion, the idea that the *T. pallidum* was not the actual causative bacterium was advanced when the influential biologist Ludwik Fleck (1896–1961) sided with Siegel and his group and when Schaudinn suddenly died from a complicated amoebic liver abscess after unsuccessful emergency surgery.[11]

By the time the famed venereologist Albert Neisser (1855–1916) initially skeptical of the spirochaete's role, had confirmed Schaudinn's work independently, it finally became official and with considerable grace Hoffman, (claiming merely to have been a collector of samples), paid honour to Schaudinn as the sole discoverer of the spirochaete as the cause of Syphilis. After this, it didn't take long for the Russian pathologist Eli Metchnikoff (1845–1916) to independently find spirochaetes lurking in the ulcers of monkeys he had inoculated with Syphilis and for others to show its presence in the livers of those children dying of congenital syphilitic disease.

---

[9] The announcement appeared as *"Vorläufiger Bericht über das Vorkommen von Spirochaeten in syphilitischen Krankheitsprodukten und bei Papillomen"*, In: *Arbeiten aus dem Kaiserlichen Gesundheitsamt*, XXII: 527–534; 25 Apr 1905.

[10] The session finished as ambiguously perhaps as it had begun with the President of the Society declaring that the session *"is closed until a new etiologic agent is found"*.

[11] Fleck became the champion of what he called the 'thought collective' (*Denkkollektiv*) which in the philosophy of science was a forerunner of Thomas Kuhn's idea of paradigmatic shift to explain the advancements in scientific thought and the way that the tenets of science (and their perceived truths) are either adopted or discarded. Fleck, despite being sent to Auschwitz Concentration Camp in 1943 and Buchenwald in 1945, survived both and between 1945 and 1952 became the head of the Institute of Microbiology at the University of Lublin. He was instrumental in establishing testing of the serologic immunologic response to syphilitic infection. Schaudinn died at the age of 35 years following emergency surgery for the parasitic infection amoebiasis which he had self-inoculated as a volunteer.

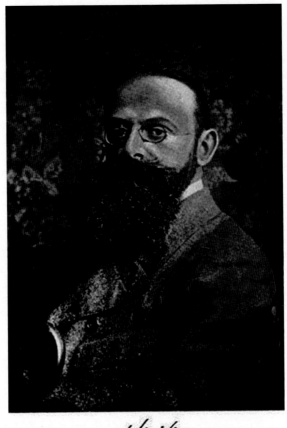

Albert Neisser (1855–1916). Wikipedia image https://en.wikipedia.org/wiki/Albert_Ludwig_
Sigesmund_Neisser

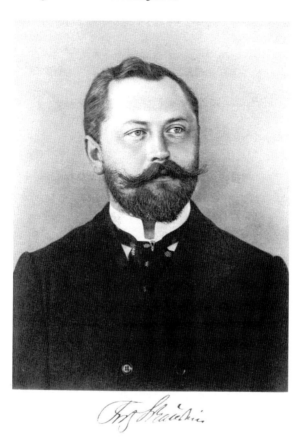

Fritz Schaudinn (1871–1906). Wikipedia https://en.wikipedia.org/wiki/Fritz_Schaudinn

Even though the culpable micro-organism had been decided upon, like other seminal diseases, the process of discovery of the causative microbe was often more a secretive than a collaborative enterprise and the vehemence of these debates sent some researchers down wasteful scientific alleyways. One of the principal investigators of Syphilis, Hideyo Noguchi (1876–1928) had by 1913 isolated the spirochaete from the brains and spinal cords of those who died either from general paresis of the insane or with the debilitating tabes dorsalis that left its victims dependent shaking cripples.[12] But Noguchi's backstory is a sad one to be sure. His demeanour as a scientist and his poor

---

[12] The work represented the staining of 70 brains with spirochaetes being detected in 14 cases. Noguchi was nominated for the Nobel Prize in 1913, 1914 and 1915, 1920, 1921 and 1924 through to 1927, however, it became increasingly clear that his work had many inaccuracies.

attention to detail ultimately resulted in tragic consequences for his collaborative team and even delayed the progress of Syphilis-related research. At the time there was greater interest in the mosquito-borne "African diseases" (yellow fever and African sleeping sickness) and the stronger imperative was to determine the cause of (and to control) an outbreak of Yellow Fever which was raging through the West Indies, Central America and Mexico and which had terrorized the gulf region of the United States.[13] As the latest epidemic had raged in Western Africa (particularly through Nigeria and Ghana) the Rockefeller Foundation deployed its most able-bodied microbiological researchers to determine if the North American and West African diseases were identical and to define the nature of the infective organism and its mechanisms of spread.

The billeting of Noguchi to coordinate the response to the epidemic proved to be disastrous. He was according to his Canadian colleague Oskar Klotz (working in Lagos and writing about Noguchi's unique laboratory manner), an irascible researcher with a remarkably slack organizational style coupled with an aggressive paranoid personality and a hair-trigger temper.[14] Noguchi's task was to catalogue the pathological material of those locally dying from Yellow Fever in West Africa and to inoculate his Rhesus monkeys with their blood and liver tissues. But his research habits were regarded as unusual, spending his working hours (which were mostly at night) in the desperate but false hope that the cause of yellow fever was the syphilitic spirocahete's relative the *leptospira icterohaemorrhagiae*. In his obsession, at any given time, Noguchi would be running and monitoring hundreds of infected monkeys alongside rooms of boxed mosquitoes (some infected and some not) with almost no notation or record of what was where. By the end, when Noguchi himself came down with a rapidly fatal case of Yellow Fever, the laboratory manager Dr William Alexander Young, (1889–1928) was lamentably forced to sweep through Noguchi's laboratory incinerating several hundred monkeys (all having been infected with trachoma virus, yellow fever and relapsing fever but with no real way of discerning which was which). Young was compelled then to fumigate the mosquito cages with cyanide gas after which he too succumbed to Yellow Fever within a days.[15]

---

[13] The concerns within the United States were quite real with cases of Yellow Fever extending in the late 1890's to endemic areas like Charleston, New Orleans and Galveston. It soon became apparent that improvements in sanitation within an inherently immune populace along with control of the breeding and migration of the mosquito population resulted in marked reductions in the number of new cases.

[14] Even by his own accounts Noguchi was not a competent pathologist. A damning analysis of Noguchi's personality and professionalism can be found in Oskar Klotz's *Diary notes on a trip to West Africa in relation to a Yellow Fever expedition under the auspices of the Rockefeller Foundation* of 1926.

[15] Noguchi had intended to flee to Africa (under the aegis of the Rockefeller Institute) after concerns had been raised regarding his research ethics injecting patients with an experimental extract from syphilitic tissue (which he called luetin) as a test to determine if there was an immunological response to prior Syphilis. The test was similar in nature to that devised by Robert Koch for the assessment of Tuberculosis activity, the Tuberculin test. But in the development of luetin, Noguchi had not sought proper informed consent from his patients and some healthy

Despite the scientific meanderings of Noguchi and his team, there was worldwide consensus that the tiny *Treponema pallidum* was the syphilitic culprit but try as they might, no one was able to take the fragile bacterium and grow it in a laboratory culture. It was stable enough to inoculate into rabbits, rodents and monkeys and there to produce some of the stages of Syphilis recognizable in humans, but no researcher could ever successfully watch it growing in a laboratory dish.[16] And so unless there was some opportunity to visualize its squirming gymnastics from the freshest of syphilitic lesions, researchers realized that they needed to diagnose the presence of the *Treponeme* by some indirect means. One of these means can be found in the blood assessing the body's immune responses once exposed to the organism. Once one has encountered the bacterium responsible for Syphilis, it leaves its immunological fingerprint, reacting to *Treponemal* invasion and multiplication by generating a raft of immune antibodies in the earliest phase of disease. These immune proteins some of which may be detected, peak in their responsiveness during the secondary stages of illness but they leave a long-term residue, (an anti-syphilitic legacy if you will), even if the *Treponeme* has in some cases been eradicated.

---

individuals ultimately acquired Syphilis. In his defence, Noguchi himself had received the injection prior to commencement of the trial but he had by that time already been diagnosed with Syphilis for which he had refused treatment. The New York Society for the Prevention of Cruelty to Children petitioned the New York District Attorney to file charges against Noguchi but the prosecution office declined. As for Young, it is likely that he contracted Yellow Fever after destroying Noguchi's laboratory although it is also possible that he could have become infected when he attended Noguchi's autopsy which had been conducted before Noguchi's remains were sent to New York.

[16] The story of the origins of the growth cultures and media which would sustain bacteria is particularly interesting and serendipitous. In the early years, Koch experimented with simple biological media in order to grow bacteria, mostly focusing on potato slices. He shifted to gelatin solutions but because he could not keep them solid at body temperature he then switched to using agar (seaweed)-impregnated dishes on the suggestion of local microbiologists Walter (1846–1911) and Fanny Hesse (1850–1934). Agar medium remains solid at body temperature (37 °C) and is transparent so that individual colonies of cultures can be observed and identified. It is also neither digested nor absorbed by most bacterial colonies. Legend has it that Frau Hesse used agar in the production of home-made jellies that she would take on picnics (as taught to her by a Dutch neighbor when Fanny was growing up in Java). Koch used the idea in his laboratories after noting that even in the heat the jelly molds didn't melt.

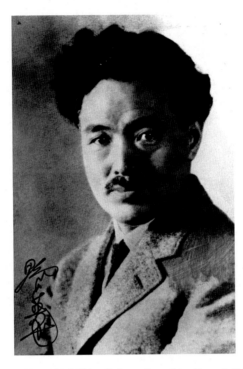

Hideyo Noguchi (1876–1928). Wikipedia https://en.wikipedia.org/wiki/Hideyo_Noguchi

The tests themselves only really show that somewhere along the journey, one has been exposed to the *Treponemal* proteins (called their antigens). They do not really tell us whether the disease is active or dormant although falling levels in specific areas (like the spinal fluid for example) at least may be a measure of treatment response. Such tests may, however, be either specific or non-specific. The principal example of one of these non-specific tests is the Wasserman reaction where serum extracted from the blood of a person exposed to Syphilis will cross-react with a similar (but surrogate) antigen that looks like a syphilitic protein.[17] One cannot overestimate the extraordinary global impact when it was introduced that this single, simple blood test had for the diagnosis of Syphilis and it made its inventor, August Paul von Wasserman (1866–1925) instantly famous.[18]

---

[17] One such commonly used protein that is a surrogate for syphilitic antigens is called cardiolipin (or Reagin). It is commercially available and is an extract of ox heart muscle (it is a complex phospholipid—diphosphatidyl glycerol). In those positive reactions, addition of the serum to the Reagin results in a visible foaming in the test tube.

[18] Subsequently, reagents for the test were mass produced at the Venereal Diseases Research Laboratory in Staten Island, New York and it became known as the VDRL test. Wasserman had developed the test in 1906 whilst working with Robert Koch and while investigating similar type tests to diagnose Tuberculosis and Diphtheria. The Wassermann test was collaborative and

Despite the fact that the genome of the *T. Pallidum* was sequenced by July 1998,[19] the science of genomics has been unable to advance our understanding of Syphilis' origin and variety. For some, the new molecular biology has provided sanctuary for novel theories of how the spirochaete has insinuated itself into the genetic fabric of Man. The biologist and Amherst Massachusetts earth mother, Lynn Margulis (1938–2011) purported that the genetic material of the spirochaete had long ago fused with the genome of the mammalian host to live in a symbiotic existence as what she had called a symbiont.[20] The new human cell with its complement of parasite DNA relied (so Margulis would have us believe) upon this commodious synergy for its own evolution and would leave new legacies. The spirocahete (she contested) had made a new and improved mammalian cell and its DNA (not ours) was the formative driving force even for the irrepressible gymnastics of sperm and also for the complexity of the interconnections of the recesses of the brain. The flagella of the spermatozoa and the dendritic ends of the neuronal cell she had felt might just share a genetic heritage with the spirochaete which long ago had bedded itself into the human cell. Her premise ambitiously placed the spirochaete front and centre in the cells that manufactured new generations and that defined the essence of our sentience as a species. We shall never know of the importance to our cells of the alien spirochaete DNA perhaps until these cell

---

included other researchers, Julius Cintron and the venereologist Albert Neisser. The group established the test for the detection of response to organisms like the *Treponeme* which could not be cultured however, these techniques have been supplanted by commercially available preparations either using purified antibodies or by DNA-based techniques to determine the presence of the Syphilis bacterium. The Wasserman test is a little unusual in the sense that if it is visualized as negative, this is suggestive of syphilitic infection. To do so it uses an indicator group of primed sheep red blood cells which (if there is no circulating antibody in the patient serum), will be destroyed leaving a small red stain. It is only where there are circulating anti-Syphilis antibodies that immune complexes will form, leaving the sheep red cells intact (so that a negative test is regarded as a positive result for Syphilis). The test uses a specialized lysing protein called complement and was one of the first blood tests using this agent and designating the test a complement-fixating test. The technique was borrowed by Wasserman from a generic complement fixation reaction first described in 1901 by Jules Bordet (1870–1961) and Octave Gengou (1875–1957). The other types of syphilis tests are more complex and involved but are specific as they examine whether the serum of an affected patient can interact directly with either a live or a killed *Treponeme* or its related generic proteins. The specifics of these tests are more relevant for those with a particular interest but include an ability of infected serum to immobilize a *Treponeme* (the *T. pallidum* immobilization test) and to interfere with its characteristic gyrations under the microscope. *Treponemal* group proteins (prepared from harmless strains such as the *T. phagadensis*) and either live or killed *T. pallidum* organisms extracted from the testicles of rabbits inoculated with the *T. pallidum* can be fixed to the surface of marker cells (like sheep or turkey red blood cells—forming the basis of the *Treponema pallidum haemagglutination* or TPHA test) or may be linked to fluorescent markers (the *Fluorescent treponemal antibody-absorption* FTA-Abs test). Molecular genetic techniques called polymerase chain reaction (pCR) which amplify the Treponemal DNA sequences have been used for difficult identification.

[19] The genome was sequenced by a collaboration between the Institute of Research Rockville Maryland and the University of Texas Health Science Center Houston.

[20] Margulis Lynn. *Symbiotic Planet: A New Look at Evolution.* Basic Books 1998.

regulators and their genetic signals can be unraveled, fingerprinted and compared, but it may explain too the tenuous connections in the neurosyphilitic between madness and genius.

Part of the history of Syphilis is the story of its treatment. It is in the traditional nature of many infective illnesses (even when their origins were still considered mysterious), that salves and medicaments will come and go in fashion. Some will be so folkloric as to acquire the sobriquet of "old wives' remedies" and others so useless that they would be the province of the quacks and the charlatans.[21] This book is not a polemic about traditional or homeopathic remedies. Nor is it one about the stories concerning the prescription of any 'little blue pills' or their advertisement through Victorian coffee houses and pie shops.[22] Even though more column space was occupied in English newspapers by anti-Syphilis medications and the parades of cures than by any other product[23] it is not too, the history of the use of the media in its pamphlets and billposters in the fight against Syphilis, although each of these topics is worthy of its own book.

Advertised discretely, Syphilis was a diagnosis which relied almost regardless of social class upon the utmost secrecy. For those attending the 18th Century physician Dr. Leveth G. West of Goose Alley in London claims of 'cures' for the "*French Distemper*" or "*a recent dose of the clap*" could be had in a matter of days "*without confinement, hindrance of business or the knowledge of a bedfellow*".[24] In this respect, some of London's Regency quacks, charging exorbitant prices for a 'cure', would even split their payments into three purses based upon the inherently

---

[21] The very idea of the 'quack' was predicated on mercuric treatments for Syphilis. Quacks or mountebanks included those using quicksilver (mercury) as part of their treatments and it is a truncation of the word 'quacksalver' which specifically targeted mercurialists. It also has origin in the Dutch word 'kwaksalver' (a hawker of salves) since Syphilis presented principally as a skin disorder but also as part of the Dutch derivation 'quacken' (a term for bragging or boasting) which was a prominent characteristic of any quacksalver.

[22] This topic is deserving of a book in itself. The Austrian Army Surgeon General Gerhard van Swieten (1700–1772) devised the ultimate use of mercuric chloride as his *Liquor Swietanii* which functioned also as a purgative; a combination ultimately superseded by Calomel (mercuric trichloride), variants of which were still available in the Australian Pharmacopoeia in 1955, the year I was born. Calomel, also known as *mercurius dulcis* or *sweet mercury* was used because of its diuretic and cathartic properties to flush the Syphilis where it was combined frequently with Opium so as to slow down absorption. There were also many regional favourites such as the *Decoctum Zitmanii* a mixture of sarsparilla root and trace elements of mercury produced by the Polish Surgeon General Friedrich Zittman (1671–1757). The most famous English 'little blue pill' for Syphilis was Dr. Leake's pills which contained a hint of mercury although they were rivalled on the Continent by the purported mercury-free preparations such as Vergery de Velnos' 'vegetable anti-venereal remedy' and the secret Laffecteur's anti-syphilitic nectar, (a likely decoction of honey, aniseed and sarsparilla root).

[23] [See Lawrence Stone. *Family Sex and Marriage in England 1500–1800*. New York Harper & Row 1972; p 600].

[24] Philip K. Wilson. *Exposing the secret disease: recognizing and treating Syphilis in Daniel Turner's London*. Ch4. In *The Secret Malady. Venereal disease in Eighteenth Century Britain and France*. Ed Linda E Merians. University Press of Kentucky 1996: pp 68–83.

secretive nature of the illness. There was a fee for the actual treatment, more money for a complete cure without fear of relapse and an additional charge for the guarantee of privacy and confidentiality.[25]

However it came into use, mercury and its variant compounds (taken internally, rubbed over the body as a luxuriant ointment, painfully injected daily or administered as an inhalable vapour across hot coals and suffumigated in specially designed absorption tents), became the mainstay of Syphilis treatment for almost 500 years.[26] How exactly it obtained its reputation for efficacy is really anyone's guess but it had been a staple in use and reserved for the swathes of medieval epidemics ranging from the Plague and leprosy by the famed surgeon Guy de Chauliac, (the personal physician to the Avignon Popes). He had written of its curative powers in his text *La Grande Chirurgie* in 1363 and the book became a manifesto for the study of anatomy and surgery in Western Europe for the next 200 years. It is likely that extensive clinical use of mercurials for Syphilis stemmed from the influential writings of Phillipus von Hohenheim (1493–1541) who came to be known by his Latin cognomen Paracelsus and whose unique brand of alchemy and mysticism would dominate the Renaissance Pharmacopoeias and establish the clan of treating 'mercurialists' and venereal disease specialists.[27] For Paracelsus (and his disciples), the ancient philosophies and their imagery were not visible in the public domain and could only be appreciated in human memory by unravelling the complex coded messages and symbolic references that permeated old manuscripts. He believed that most illnesses could be ameliorated by chemical means specifically through the use of treatment with combinations of metallic compounds. But his prolific writings aimed to combine allegory and science and they influenced many writers and philosophers.[28] For Paracelsus, cryptically he would remark *"that which lives on reason lives against the spirit"* advocating the need to follow the premise of the Third Empire of the Holy Spirit where all that was literal and evident would be replaced by an holistic understanding of the meaning of the great texts and where the essence of the Universe would be revealed to believers in a Great

---

[25] See Daniel Turner. *The Modern quack (or the physical impostor detected)* 1718 cited by WF Bynum. In *Treating the wages of sin: venereal disease and specialism in Eighteenth Century Britain*. In *Medical Fringe and Medical Orthodoxy* 1750–1850. WF Bynum and Roy Porter (Eds). London Croom Helm 1987.

[26] As metallic mercury is so poorly absorbed, it was administered either as an unguant or as a vapour. Fumigation tents for Syphilis treatment, (begun in the 16th Century), were continued in use up until the 1920's. [See Goldwater LJ. *Mercury: a history of quicksilver*. Baltimore York Press 1972].

[27] Paracelsus was also known by the extraordinarily whimsical title Theophrastus Bombastus von Hohenheim.

[28] William Blake (1757–1827) was an ardent admirer of this theosophic approach believing that *"every age renews its powers from these works"* (quoted from his poem *Jerusalem*, verse 60). The complex literary cross-referencing found in the writings of Paracelsus also influenced the works of Yeats, Joyce and Rimbaud, the philosophy of Hegel and some of the treatises of the psychoanalyst Carl Jung. [See also Alexander Roob. *Alchemy and Mysticism*. Taschen1997].

Book.[29] His prolific work set out detailed instructions for the manufacture of a range of pharmaceutical remedies (based on an understanding of plants and metals) that cross-referenced to an overarching prophesy concerning the arts of magic derived from a unique fusion of Jewish Kabbalistic texts, Christian (and Pre-Christian) mysticism and astrological charts. It was (at least in its beginnings) perhaps the strangest basis for the chemical treatment of Syphilis.

Even without a clear understanding of the cause of Syphilis, Fracastoro's influence too on the proposed methods of contagion had proven so persuasive that mercury, (which induced copious salivation and sweating during its treatment use), was thought to leech the offending 'virus' of Syphilis and simply flush it out. In short, the higher the tolerable mercury dose and the more sweat and saliva it produced during treatment, the better.[30] There is no doubt that the cure for some proved worse than the disease and both came with deserved reputations. But the approach was philosophical too. Prior to the discovery by Schaudinn and Hoffmann of the causative bacterium, Syphilis was something that medications could only eliminate from the body. The finding of a discrete cause for the disease induced the search for a new type of compound, a magic bullet capable of annihilating the culpable microorganism.

Far from the anonymity and privacy that might be gained by ingesting unmarked pills (some of which were even covered in chocolate coating to hide the indication for their use), the litany of mercury's side-effects, most notably the loss of hair, the

---

[29] The Third Empire of the Holy Spirit which guided Paracelsus had been foretold by the theologian Joachim of Fiore (1135–1202) after an epiphany he (i.e. Joachim) had experienced travelling in Jerusalem. It had prophesied the mechanism whereby Man would come into direct contact with God and Joachim was considered so important that King Richard the Lionheart sought a meeting with Joachim before embarking on the 3rd Crusade.

[30] Here there are numerous accounts of complicated protocols and rituals in the use of the mercury friction rub. The London physician Daniel Turner had a rigorous régime rubbing the feet only over the first day and then over a week gradually progressing up to the buttocks and the genitals. This would be associated with food restriction (except for the ingestion of a small poached egg) swaddling the patient in thick blankets and placing them in front of a roaring open fire to induce between 2 and 3 pints (as measured) of saliva daily. The hypersalivation (known as *ptyalism*) was believed to be particularly excessive with mercury-sulphur combinations (prescribed as Cinnabar) thought to possess both magical and astrological powers. [See Debus AG. *The Chemical Philosophy and Alchemy Book*. New York Science History Publications 1977: 80–4]. Mercury was medicinally available in a range of less toxic preparations including bromides, nitrates and as sulphides. Another commonly used variant was a combination of mercuric dichloride, copper sulphate and salt which was called 'corrosive sublimate' and which was the principal agent used as a fumigant or mixed usually with hog's fat to be topically applied to the skin. Paracelsus using a combination of gold, mercury and cinnabar devised as his '*elixir vitae*' which he considered a cure for both Syphilis and leprosy.

discolouration, rotting and falling out of the teeth and an incessant shaking were publicly visible enough giveaways to those with any social knowledge of the disease to determine that someone was undergoing mercury treatment.[31] But despite the greatest show of secrecy concerning one's management, (particularly amongst the aristocracy), the visibility of facial ulceration and the tremulous palsy would not require much sleuthing and few would need to be any sort of detective to have figured out the cause for a local Laird's mental and physical deterioration.

Syphilis had single-handedly demarcated the medical professions. The physicians, (specialists of medicine) could look after all that was occult and internal (hence internists) whilst the surgeons dealt with the exterior visible ravages of disease. And so the vast work of venereal disease was the province of the surgeons, free to drain venereal abscesses and buboes, to cauterize chancres, rub down verrucous and contagious warts and to lance carbuncles and pustules. If mercury then was one side of the treating fence, on the other side there were the staunch 'anti-mercurialists'. Perhaps the earliest of these was Ulrich von Hutten whose syphilitic woes he attested were eased more greatly by his guiacum wood brought from the forests of Hispañola than by any mercurial rubbing. But his exhortations were not well received, more likely because as a Benedictine monk he had been so staunchly pro-Lutheran and had on more than one occasion suffered the rebukes of Pope Leo X. It had forced Ulrich into exile on the island of Ufenau in Lake Zurich where he wrote incessantly about the terrible dental decay he had experienced at the hands of his treating surgeons.[32] Mercury treatments particularly as a series of painful injections, had provoked so much toxicity that the subject generated its own 'industry' with Johann Karl Proksch (1840–1923), a noted medical historian

---

[31] The use of a range of inorganic mercuric salts induces peripheral nerve damage with in some, florid symptoms suggesting that worms are crawling under the skin (*formication* as it is called). Some of the neurological dysfunction observed mimicked the symptoms of neurosyphilis and it was, in the absence of any discrete diagnostic tests, impossible to distinguish between the two. Shaking of the hands (with an impairment in handwriting that characteristically looped words on top of one another) coupled with an emotional shyness were particular features of mercury poisoning.

[32] This particular side-effect of mercury treatment was also a concern for Oscar Wilde. Wilde's biographer Robert Sherrard reprinted some of an earlier biographer Boris Brasol's assertions that Wilde had Syphilis and that his mercury injections had resulted in "*Wilde's teeth* [growing] *black and* [which] *became decayed.*" [See Boris Brasol. *Oscar Wilde: The Man, the Artist, the Martyr.* New York Octagon 1975; p 384. Quoted in Hayden. *Ibid.* p 208].

writing five scathing volumes on the matter.[33] According to the British ophthal-
mologist John O'Shea, the 19th Century saw over 3000 medical articles released on
Syphilis treatment.[34] Of these, one-third were devoted to mercurial remedies and
fully one-tenth just to its toxic reactions.

Severe problems with the old methods of treatment spurred on researchers to
find new compounds that would cure Syphilis without actually killing their patients,
but the enthusiasm of some would give way to a deficient ethical standard of care in
the manner in which they experimented upon their cases; a story examined in
Chap. 6 of this book. The lock hospital wards in London along with many country
mansions were filled with victims engaged in the 'salivating cure' and it resulted in
the confusion of so many cases presenting with a perverse mimicry of the neurologic disorder the treatments were designed to assuage. In this cycle the arrival by
1910 of the arsenical compounds through the tireless animal experimentation of
Paul Ehrlich (1854–1915) and the preliminary results on four young men with early
Syphilis treated with the wonder drug Penicillin by a team headed by John
Mahoney at the Staten Island Venereal Diseases Research Laboratory in 1943,
would both prove to be convulsive events in the history of the disease. With both of
these new chemicals, venereal disease conferences would herald the breakthrough
as the beginning of the end of the syphilitic microorganism, [35] but on each occasion

---

[33] JK Proksch. *Die Geshgite da Verorische Krankheiten.* Bonn Peter Hanstein 1895. Columbia
University's Emeritus Professor of Medicine Leonard Goldwater (1903–1992) in his book
Mercury—a History of Quicksilver (Baltimore York Press 1972) perhaps overstated it when he
wrote "*the use of mercury in the treatment of syphilis may have been the most colossal hoax ever
perpetrated in a profession which has never been free of hoaxes*".

[34] JG O'Shea. *Two minutes with Venus, two years with mercury. Mercury as an anti-syphilitic
chemotherapeutic agent.* Journal of the Royal Society of Medicine 1990; 83: 392–6. O'Shea
contests that the violinist Niccolò Paganini (1782–1840) was poisoned with mercury after a
presumptive diagnosis of Syphilis by his attending physician Dr. Sira Borda. [See JG O'Shea. *Was
Paganini poisoned with mercury?* Journal of the Royal Society of Medicine 1988; 81: p 594–7].

[35] The history of anti-Syphilis treatment breakthroughs has always been one which has falsely
prophesied the total eradication of the spirochaete. In 1948, President Harry S. Truman set up a
committee of the Department of Defense chaired by the then President of the National Social
Welfare Assembly, Frank Weil to eradicate Syphilis by a concerted abstinence (over condom use)
as part of a National strategy. The CDC reiterated the desire to 'eradicate venereal disease' in a
formal manifesto in 1972 but the year would see the CDC embroiled in the ethical controversy of
its direct involvement in denying Tuskegee Alabaman African Americans with proven latent
Syphilis any form of antibacterial therapy (see Chap. 6).

as the claim would ring out that Syphilis had been defeated, the wily spirochaete would somehow persist and prevail.[36]

It is perhaps timely to divert a little in order to consider the life of Ehrlich. Although he was awarded the Nobel Prize in 1908 more for his conceptual work on the immune system, he will always be remembered for his meticulous approach towards finding a chemical cure for both Syphilis and African sleeping sickness.[37] He was at one and the same time both a complex and a simple man, driven by a self-imposed routine, writing out his daily laboratory instructions on small coloured pieces of paper and content to carry out his research in a tiny laboratory crammed to the rafters with notes and documents. It was pain of death to disturb them and like all busy eccentrics, he could instantaneously lay his hands on anything amongst the chaos of papers. By all accounts he displayed a remarkable generosity and although a little intolerant of fools, he could be extraordinarily patient. His fame became so great that he would speak at many international meetings in now a broken English or sometimes in a fractured French. Even his native German was described as 'simple' and although his lectures were well received, they were never as of such great moment as the conceptual ideas he proposed. In short, he was the father (indeed even the inventor) of our understanding of human antibodies and of the basis of the immune system and he was the first to suggest that cancers might be controlled chemically by interruption of their cell cycle or their protein machinery.

---

[36] Before the advent of Ehrlich's arsenic cures for Syphilis, the English surgeon William Wallace (1791–1837) had introduced potassium iodide which was moderately effective particularly when mixed with small quantities of mercury to reduce toxicity coupled with concoctions of other metals which frequently included tellurium, vanadium, platinum and gold. Bismuth for the treatment of Syphilis sufferers was introduced in 1884 as a less toxic alternative with an ability to kill the spirochaete (what was referred to as spirilocidal activity). Its clinical use in Europe was advanced by Robert Sazerac, Constantin Levaditi and Louis Fournier. Bismuth was effective against the cutaneous syphilide lesions and sporadically resulted in sufficient spirochaete death as to render those cases with secondary syphilis non-infectious.

[37] The Nobel Prize was awarded jointly to Ehrlich and Eli Metchnikoff for his discovery of the immune scavenging cell the macrophage and its cellular mechanism of ingesting bacteria (which he had called phagocytosis). The initial Nobel Prizes were in the hands of a committee of physicians at the Karolinska Institute whose task it was to consider nominations and write position papers on candidates discussing their pros and cons so that decisions were in the hands of a few powerful judges. Notification of the Faculty committee to the Nobel Committee was then made orally. Debate centred around the spirit of Alfred Nobel's will which was unclear concerning whether the prize could be awarded for past work or only for more recent research. The expectation was that the research or work had either benefitted mankind or had the potential to do so. Ehrlich was nominated once in 1901 (but lost in the inaugural prize to Emil von Behring). He was nominated twice in both 1902 and 1903, nine times in 1904, seven times in 1905, nine times in 1906, seventeen times in 1907 and twelve times the year he won it in 1908. After his laureateship, he was nominated for a second prize some 22 more times. [See Ulf Lagerkvist. *Pioneers of Microbiology and the Nobel Prize*. World Scientific New Jersey 2003; pp. 111–124, 141–171].

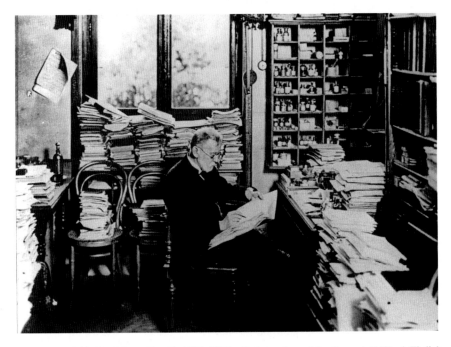

Paul Ehrlich in his Frankfurt office Ca 1900. Wikipedia https://en.wikipedia.org/wiki/Paul_Ehrlich

In her soft epitaph affectionately collated by his devoted secretary Martha Marquhardt there is a striking naivete in her writing.[38] She seemed incredulous after working with Ehrlich for so many years to find out that he was proudly Jewish. It had held up some of his appointments and when he had commenced work with the microbiologist Robert Koch, Ehrlich continued in Koch's laboratory for three years unpaid.[39] With her Prussian upbringing that had cemented the exclusion of Jews from so many areas of academia, all Marquhardt could say on the matter was her impression that "*he* [i.e. Ehrlich] *would never have thought of changing his religion for the sake of deriving any advantage by so doing*".[40] It was a remarkable misunderstanding (even though Jews could be offered ceremonial baptisms), by someone purportedly closest to him of the meaning of Ehrlich's secular sense of Jewishness. What irony it was that her earlier book on Ehrlich, *Paul Ehrlich als Mensch und Arbeiter* (Paul Ehrlich, the Man and his Work) written in 1924 was subsequently banned and destroyed by the Nazis.

---

[38] Martha Marquhardt, (Ehrlich's secretary for 15 years until his death in 1915) wrote a loving biography in 1949. *Paul Ehrlich.* Introduction by Sir Henry Dale. William Heinemann Medical Books Ltd 1949.

[39] As a Jew, Ehrlich's position as Professor at Berlin University was also nominal. His laboratory expenses were ultimately covered by a personal grant from the wealthy Frankfurt, von Speyer family (the George-Speyer Haus for Chemotherapy. The grant was organized by Speyer's widow Franziska).

[40] Marquhardt. *Ibid.* p. 160.

Like many geniuses, Ehrlich came from humble beginnings and there is little in his early life to intimate any particular greatness. Born in Strehlen (near Breslau in what is now Poland but then was part of Prussia), his abiding love of chemistry was instilled in him by his grandfather who ran a chemical plant.[41] Ehrlich was a particularly sensitive man and decided to devote himself to laboratory activities rather than patient care. It would cost him dearly in sponsorship and he would always be beholden to personal benefactors for research support.[42] His 1877 doctorate thesis had even found a new blood cell, (the mast cell), identifiable through its azure blue staining. It would be designated later as an initiating cell of allergic responses.[43]

Collaborating with Emil von Behring, (1854–1917) he standardized diphtheria anti-toxin for immunization showing how to enhance its production by injecting it into horses. But the mass production of antibodies created a personal rift between the two men over the financial arrangements and Ehrlich always felt excluded and somewhat betrayed.[44] By 1904, Ehrlich had established his first Japanese collaboration with Kiyoshi Shiga (1871–1957) again staining cells infected with the African sleeping sickness Trypanosomiasis and showing that the agent Trypan red could neutralize the parasite.[45] More importantly, Ehrlich was the first to show benefit from an arsenic-based compound Atoxyl and although some cases suffered the serious side-effect of blindness with its use, Ehrlich became convinced that Arsenical compounds would change the way such diseases could be treated.[46] Convinced of the

---

[41] As a child Ehrlich developed an interest in dyes and vital stains of tissues which formed the basis of his work with aniline compounds that stained the recently discovered Mycobacterium bacillus responsible for Tuberculosis. His specialized technique brought him to the attention of Robert Koch and was the forerunner of Ehrlich's side-chain theory of chemical attraction. Ehrlich became so enamored with chemical dyes that as a young boy he spiked the feed of his parents' pigeons with an aniline compound in the hope that they would turn purple. Unaware of its inherent toxicity, he was disappointed to find all of them dead the next day.

[42] Ehrlich worked under the auspices of Friedrich Althoff (1839–1908) of the Prussian Department of Education and earlier in Berlin's Charité Hospital under its benevolent Medical Director Friedrich Theodor von Frerichs (1819–1885). Von Frerichs gave Ehrlich free reign to pursue his researches, a privilege rescinded after von Frerichs tragically committed suicide.

[43] MD Thesis P Ehrlich. *Some Constituents to the Theory and Praxis of Histological Staining.* 1877. Ehrlich's early work also categorized white blood cells based upon staining techniques which are still in essence used today. He was also the first to classify leukemias by their inherent cell type.

[44] Afterwards, both men were isolated and they remained only poorly reconciled. Ehrlich never shared in von Behring's financial success with Diphtheria antitoxin production. It has been estimated that von Behring's share in the profits made by Fabwerke Hoechst between 1895 and 1914 were around 1,847,000 Marks (about 30 Million DM in today's exchange). [Quoted by Witkop *Ibid.* p. 551 and also by Throm Carola. *Das Diphtherie Serum in Wissenschatliche Verlagsgessellschaft* Stuttgart 1995.

[45] There had always been a fascination by European researchers at the turn of the 19th Century with this African parasitic disease transmitted by the bite of the exotic Tse-Tse fly particularly following a devastating epidemic in Uganda in 1901 which claimed 250,000 people.

[46] Pre-empting Schaudinn's discovery of the spirochaete, after showing a colleague a specimen jar containing a syphilitic chancre, Ehrlich was quoted as saying "*when the microbe causing syphilis is found, I must be prepared*". Quoted in A Lennox Thorburn. *Paul Ehrlich: pioneer of chemotherapy and cure by arsenic (1854–1915).* British Journal of Venereal Diseases 1983; 59: pp. 404–5. The compound

importance of these Arsenicals, Ehrlich now supported by his most meticulous and obsessive coworker Sahachiro Hata, (1873–1938) methodically and painstakingly examined hundreds of arsenic-based agents in animals to attest whether they would attenuate the progression of Syphilis. Of these, by the fourth year of study with the 606th chemical assessed, (an arsenobenzene compound called Arsphenamine) he had finally shown a resilient ability to control the disease in rabbits (as well as to ameliorate relapsing fever in his mice and rats). The 606 agent was so useful that he quickly re-named it Salvarsan and set about placing it into heavy production after officially announcing its success at the Congress for Internal Medicine on April 19th 1910 in Wiesbaden. After that meeting, for almost the rest of the year Ehrlich was mobbed at any conference and usually arrived with a police escort.

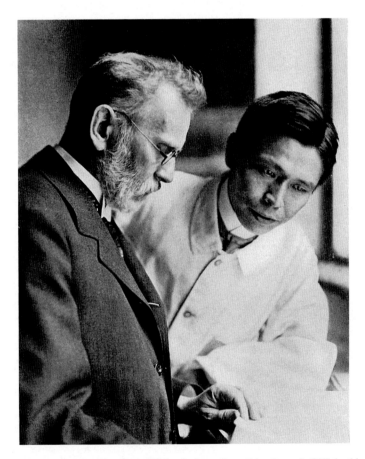

Ehrlich with coworker Sahachiro Hata. Wikipedia https://en.wikipedia.org/wiki/Sahachiro_Hata

---

Atoxyl (p-aminophenylarsonic acid) was developed in collaboration with Alfred Bertheim and then once found to be effective against Syphilis, produced on an industrial scale.

There should be little debate concerning the global impact of 606 as despite the fact that it needed to be administered by daily painful injection and also possessed some severe side-effects, it changed Syphilis management almost overnight and drew the attention of the Nobel Committee. Thomas Edison, when asked by the Hearst Press to define the most significant events of the previous year, remarked that *"along with the political idea that China should be transformed into a republic, it* [Salvarsan] *was the second greatest event of 1910"*.[47] Demand for 606 was so great that Ehrlich produced the first 65,000 doses with the Hoechst Company through a complicated final anaerobic step that vacuum sealed the glass ampoules for distribution from his Speyer Haus Frankfurt laboratories. All doses were released free of charge to researchers around the world.

But there was trouble ahead that would take its physical toll on Ehrlich. Whether it was jealousy, or anti-Semitism, who would know but a street ascetic taken to dressing up as a monk Karl Wassman, the editor of the magazine *Der Freigeist, (The Libertine)* had become incensed with the way Salvarsan was being administered.[48] In a public lawsuit naming Ehrlich and his clinical coordinator Karl Herxheimer (1861–1942),

---

[47] Hata had been sent to Ehrlich's laboratory from Tokyo's Kitasato Institute for Infectious Diseases after Ehrlich had read of Hata's ability to grow the syphilitic spirochaete in rabbits. When Hata arrived he was initially asked to compare the efficacy of Compound No. 418 with Compound No. 606. Both Ehrlich and Hata were obsessively organized and they went on to retest almost all of the 600 available compounds in the new animal model. The compound 606 (dihydroxy-diaminoarsenobenze) was precipitated as a salt with hydrochloric acid. Edison thought Salvarsan was even more important than any recent advances in aerial navigation. Edison's comments if not overly specific, were a humbling admission by a man whose life was predicated on the secrecy and intrigues of independent discovery and who himself was viscerally anti-Semitic. [Edison quote from the *San Francisco Examiner* January 3rd 1912. Also See Henry F. May. *The End of American Innocence: A Study of the First Years of Our Own Time, 1912–1917*. New York Columbia University Press. 1992; p. 14–15]. Ehrlich's colleague Albert Neisser initially skeptical of the benefit of arsenic was by the end, emphatic. *"606"* he wrote *"whatever the future may bring is now more or less an incredible advance."* [See Benedek TG. Albert Neisser 1855–1916. Microbiologist and Venereologist at http://www. antimicrobe.org/h04c.files/history/Neisser.asp.

[48] Wassmann's magazine was variably also entitled, '*The Truth*,' '*Love*' and '*The Free Spirit*'.

Wassman asserted that as a treatment, it was unnatural, poisonous and coercive. Ehrlich was shocked and determined as a very private man not to attend the proceedings, only reluctantly testifying at the end so as to defend his prized discovery and its legacy. It was a particularly public and personal form of attack. The accusations that he had profited through his shares with the Hoechst Pharmaceutical Company were particularly hurtful and he was forced to take out pages in the *München Medizinischen Wochenschrift* journal to refute the claims. The article in a medical journal ignominiously included tabulated proof that Ehrlich had channelled profits directly back into the Speyer Haus research laboratory rather than pocketing them for his own gain. Even claims that he had bought a brand-new town car had to be refuted in the public press. Worse too for Ehrlich was a rogue clinic in Prague that had reported fatal neurological and kidney problems after Salvarsan's use, resulting in an overall death rate from the wonder drug of about 1 in every 1000 people treated.[49]

As for Wassmann, he was convicted of libel and sentenced to a year in prison, two months only of which he served following the general amnesty of inmates at the start of World War 1. Herxheimer was not so lucky. After the Nazi ascension to power, they ensured that he could not work in his Frankfurt Clinic and he was deported to Thieresenstadt concentration camp where he perished. Ehrlich, exhausted after the trial first endured one stroke and then another and passed away whilst taking a resting cure at Bad Homburg. He never really recovered from the stress and was unable to realize his passionate dream to establish Europe's first Institute for Vital Staining.[50]

---

[49] Ehrlich was convinced that the deaths from Salvarsan were due to faulty preparation and deviation from his strict method of storage. Another critic of Ehrlich was Victor Mentberger from the University of Strasbourg who chronicled in his deposition the lethality of Compound 606. Ehrlich's 'chemical' response to criticisms regarding the toxicity of Salvarsan was to get his colleague Bertheim to produce a soluble variant which they called Neo-Salvarsan, but it was never as efficacious.

[50] Ehrlich had written to Professor William Welch in Baltimore about this new Institute in January 1915. He had always anticipated that it would be directed by his star pupil, Freiberg's Professor Goldman but with Goldman's sudden death in 1914, the outbreak of the War and Ehrlich's illness, the plans came to nothing.

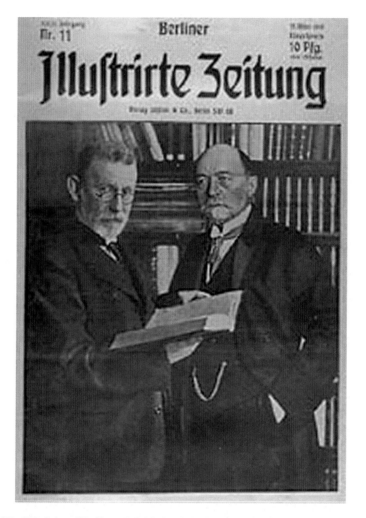

Image of Paul Ehrlich and Emil von Behring in 1914 when the two Nobel laureates both celebrated their 60th birthdays (Ehrlich was born on March 14th and von Behring on March 15th). Although von Behring gave the eulogy at Ehrlich's funeral, the two men were estranged so that the title page of the Berliner Illustrierten Zeitung suggesting a happy relationship was only the result of a photomontage of 2 pre-existing individual photos

The Nobel Committee then turned its attention to a little known Austrian psychiatrist, Julius Wagner-Jauregg (1857–1940)[51] who had noted that patients with neurosyphilis became improved after they had experienced high fevers. He became

---

[51] He was born Julius Wagner but his family name was changed to Wagner von Jauregg after his father Adolph was conferred an hereditary Austro-Hungarian Empire title in 1883 going under the name Julius Wagner Ritter von Jauregg. After dissolution of the Empire at the close of 1918 he contracted his name to Wagner-Jauregg.

excited by this idea of 'pyrotherapy' and began inoculating his patients with malaria after first failing to successfully inoculate them with bacteria (mostly streptococci in culture) or Robert Koch's tuberculosis extract, Tuberculin.[52] The theory behind this was that the *Treponema pallidum* organism of Syphilis was heat intolerant (what is referred to as heat labile) and that in higher temperature environments it would simply die. The malaria, Wagner-Jauregg had said could readily be treated with some Quinine.[53] The improvements reported with the treatment exceeded 50% in some studies and for a short time malaria therapy spread across Europe and into the United States.[54] Reporting on one case of a 37 year-old actor rendered a vegetable with General Paresis of the Insane, after a year of treatment Wagner-Jauregg triumphantly declared that the young man had happily returned to the stage. The Nobel Committee recommended Wagner-Jauregg for the 1927 Prize and in the introduction of the laureate Professor W. Wernstedt, Dean of the Royal Caroline Institute in Sweden had remarked on the philosophy that *"one must expel evil with evil"*.[55] In retrospect, the Nobel Committee can occasionally get it wrong. If evil there was, others had shown that the response was just as great to a hyperthermic cabinet that would raise the bodily core temperature without the malarial risk. The

---

[52] Although Koch was awarded the Grand Cross of the Order of the Red Eagle for discovery of a glycerine extract from the Mycobacterium (which he called Tuberculin) his reputation took a severe blow after it proved a clinical failure in Tuberculosis prevention and treatment.

[53] Wagner-Jauregg had been stimulated to malaria use after personally meeting a soldier returning from the Macedonian front in 1917 who was infected with Tertian malaria (which induces fevers every 3 nights). His technique was to take the blood from such patients at the height of their fever and then inject it in small quantity just under the skin between the shoulder blades of his neurosyphilis cases. When they would experience fever this would be secondarily treated with Quinine. Although his intention was to inoculate his patients with the more innocuous protozoal type of malaria called *Plasmodium vivax*, he inadvertently injected the more virulent strain *Plasmodium Falciparum* into some patients and three of them died.

[54] Malaria therapy was used up until the 1920's in Denmark for example extending its prescription for psychotic patients. Its use raised serious ethical concerns regarding the nature of informed consent triggering a National debate. [See Kragh, Jesper Vaczy. *Malaria fever therapy for General Paresis of the Insane in Denmark*. History of Psychiatry 2010; 21: pp. 1–6]. For the use of Malaria therapy in the United States See Grob GN. *The Mad Among Us: A History of the Care of America's Mentally Ill*. New York Free Press 1994 and also Braslow J. *Mental Ills and Bodily Cures: Psychiatric treatment in the first half of the 20th Century*. Berkeley University of California Press 1997].

[55] Address delivered December 10th 1927. Quoted from Nobel Lectures, Physiology and Medicine 1922–1941 Elsevier Publications Amsterdam 2965. Copyrights Nobel Foundation. Reprinted from Wagner-Jauregg's original article: Verhutung und Behandlung der progressiven Paralyse durch Impfmalaria (Prevention and treatment of progressive paralysis by malaria inoculation). Printed in the 1931 Memorial Volume of the Handbuch der experimentellen Therapie.

technique with all its attendant ethical woes gradually fell out of favour particularly since as many as 15% of patients had died during therapy. After this Wagner-Jauregg himself fell out of favour with his openly anti-Semitic displays. Even though Austria's Nazi Party (the NSDAP) refused him membership because his first wife Balbine Frumkin was Jewish, Wagner-Jauregg to prove his party loyalty became a strong advocate for the eugenic control of what he regarded as the inferior races. He ended life administering thyroid hormones and ovarian preparations to prepubescent youths and sterilizing some psychotic patients in an attempt so he declared, to stop them masturbating.

As much of an advance as Salvarsan was, it was a complex drug to produce and administer requiring a prolonged series of painful and sometimes toxic injections. More than this, its value in latent and tertiary Syphilis associated with organ damage was uncertain. The new breakthrough, Penicillin, discovered in 1929 by Alexander Fleming (1881–1955), changed Syphilis forever even though it failed to eradicate it worldwide. For Fleming, Penicillin was a drug of potential but for his co-worker Howard Florey (1898–1968) and also for Oxford's Ernst Chain (1906–1979) the challenge was its mass production.[56] Before it had even shown efficacy against Syphilis, the US Army in collaboration with the Pfizer Company (which had set up a mass scale production unit in Brooklyn New York), was shipping it out to the European War Theatre where it had already shown responses against staphylococcal and streptococcal wound infections in the field.[57]

---

[56] Heavy production of Penicillin hinged on some rather small fortuitous events. Florey saw the need to move production to the United States in the summer of 1941 and together with Norman Heatley visited the Northern Research Laboratory in Peoria Illinois translating lessons learned from agricultural fermentation into industrial mould culture. Their Director Orville May taught Florey how to increase production by adding corn-steep liquor to the culture and medical historian John Parascandola recounts that the most active *Penicillium* strain was obtained from a mouldy canteloupe bought at the Peoria fruit market. [See John Parascandola. John Mahoney and the introduction of Penicillin to treat Syphilis. Presented as a paper at the History of Pharmacy Congress Florence, Italy October 20th to 23rd 1999].

[57] The War Production Bond initiated national manufacture of Penicillin under the Directorship of Albert Elder so that sufficient antibiotics would be available for the D-Day landings. [See Albert L. Elder. *The history of Penicillin production.* New York. American Institute of Chemical Engineers. 1970].

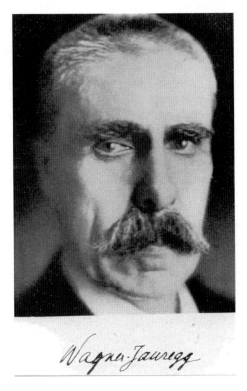

Julius Wagner-Jauregg (1857–1940) Wikipedia: https://en.wikipedia.org/wiki/Julius_Wagner-Jauregg

In the United States by 1919, the Chamberlain-Kahn Act had instituted a Division of Venereal Diseases section within the Public Health Service (PHS)[58] with its other provisions permitted the allocation of federal funds to the states on designated projects. The Surgeon General at the time Thomas Parran Jr (1892–1968) invited the new Director of the Venereal Diseases Research Laboratory (the VDRL) John Friend Mahoney (1889–1957) to establish a combined research facility and clinical treatment station in Staten Island New York.[59] Mahoney's brief was the examination of the ability of the spirochaete to penetrate tissues but his

---

[58] The Chamberlain-Kahn Act was registered by Congress in July 1918 as An Act Making Appropriations for the Support of the Army for the Fiscal year ending June 30th 1919, detaining and quarantining 20,000 women as a public health measure. The Act established a National Social Hygiene Board which included the Secretary of War, the Secretary of the Navy and the Secretary of the Treasury, the Surgeon General of the Army and the Navy and the Surgeon General of the Public Health Service as sitting members.

[59] At the time, rabbit experiments with Syphilis were already being conducted at the PHS Hygiene Laboratory (which was the forerunner of the National Institutes of Health—the NIH) and clinical studies on Syphilis were underway in Hot Springs Arkansas.

secondary aim was to determine the efficacy of the new antibiotic, Sulfonamide in a commoner US Army problem, gonorrhoea. The first trials of Penicillin conducted by Mahoney and his colleague R.C. Arnold against spirochaetes proved singularly disappointing and under normal circumstances that may have ended there. But Mahoney tried again on his syphilitic rabbits figuring that the new drug was largely non-toxic and if it didn't work he could always rely on Salvarsan. By June 1943, he had treated and reported 4 human patients with early Syphilis giving them daily injections of Penicillin intramuscularly for a week with complete eradication of the disease on follow-up.

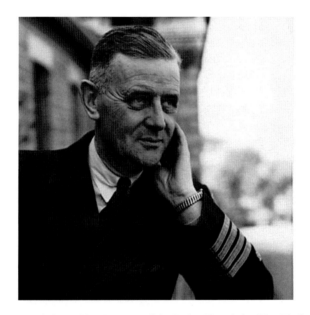

John Friend Mahoney (1889–1957) Courtesy of the Lasker Foundation New York. He ultimately became New York City's Commissioner of Health in 1950

After an inauspicious start to his presentation at the American Public Health Association on October 14th, the response of the gathering was electric.[60] Mahoney himself was stunned by the audience reaction but immediately realized the need for further testing as there were in his mind so many unanswered questions. What was the optimal dose? How long should patients be treated for? How would Penicillin interact with other drugs? Will it treat tertiary forms of the disease? All of this would be rapidly sorted once the turmoil had settled down and the hard graft of

[60] One microbiologist at the meeting Gladys Hobby writing her account of Mahoney's presentation, recalled that she couldn't contain her excitement. [See Gladys Hobby. *Penicillin. Meeting the Challenge*. New Have CT Yale University Press. 1985].

science took over.[61] Cooler heads prevailed in the scientific community as the *New York Times* declared on the 26th May 1944 the *"End of Syphilis seen by Use of Penicillin"* and as the *Chicago Tribune* heralded on February 6th 1946 that soon enough *"everyone would be on it."* Reactions ran from a relieved public to puritanical wowsers warning that Penicillin would only lead to widespread promiscuity and encourage the disease it was designed (albeit fortuitously) to prevent. Penicillin would be so effective that sometimes upon its use, high fevers would be endured with the mass death of the spirochaetes, lurking in previously immune areas of the body. Patients although improving would shiver and shake as large numbers of bacteria would release their protein products from the hidden sanctums that had previously defied treatment. The response (called the Jarisch–Herxheimer reaction)[62] became so characteristic that some had warned that Penicillin should be denied as treatment to those with latent disease and it had been used as an excuse by the Alabama state doctors to prevent the care of African American men, just to see how Syphilis 'behaved' if untreated. Lumbering philosophies too would try and catch up with burgeoning science and struggle to come to terms with medicine's presumptive invincibility. Overconfident, by 1953 the Eisenhower Administration convinced of a superiority over the infection unsuccessfully proposed eliminating the VDRL altogether.[63]

---

[61] JR Heller Jr (1905–1989) the Head of the VD Division of the PHS between 1943 and 1948 wrote of Penicillin " *overshadowing anything that has happened in Syphilis control since the days of Ehrlich.*" [See JR Heller Jr. *Syphilis control in wartime.* Southern Medical Journal 1944; 37: pp. 219–223].

[62] The Jarisch–Herxheimer reaction can also occasionally be seen during the treatment of other spirochaetal infections such as Lyme disease and relapsing fever as well as in leptospirosis and a parrot-transmitted infestation Q fever (psittacosis). It is also seen in some infectious conditions specifically affecting the brain, most notably trichinosis (tapeworm infestation) and trypanosomiasis (African sleeping sickness).

[63] See John Parascandola. Ch. 6. *Magic in the form of Penicillin: Syphilis in America since World War II.* In J Parascandola. *Sex Sin and Science. A History of Syphilis in America.* Praeger Westport 2008: pp. 133–154.

Chapter 5
Notable Victimhood: Syphilis and the Arts

We all have the republican spirit in our veins, like syphilis in our bones. We are democratized and venerealized
Charles Baudelaire (1821–1867)

Abstract Despite its ubiquitous presence, Syphilis was no great inspiration for authors. It settled in Larry Tighe the protagonist of Rudyard Kipling's *The Love-o'-Women*. But it had also settled in the brains of Baudelaire and Flaubert and in the mind of de Maupassant who thought its presence the source of his great genius. The Romanian philosopher and ardent Francophile Emil Cioran yearned for its infection if only to be blessed with the visitation of a syphilitic muse. The artistic legacy of Syphilis lay in the face of Rembrandt's favourite pupil Gerard de Lairesse whose coarse features, his saddle nose, bossed forehead and thick lips are textbook traits of a congenital syphilitic. The images of the Belgian artist Félicien Rops show Syphilis as a deadly temptress holding the scythe of the Grim Reaper (*La Faucheuse*).

The world of Syphilis, (although accruing many illustrious victims), has never really engendered the great repository of reverent literature comparable to that which has chronicled the last terminal gasps of Tuberculosis or the ravages of the Black Death. Syphilis was unable to bring forth the romance of the consumptive poet John Keats (1795–1821) repeatedly haemorrhaging from his lungs in 1820 that left him weakened even further when his physicians felt that the only treatment was to bleed him more. His final weeks would be unassuaged by a desperate trip to enjoy the soothing climate of Rome.[1] Nor could it evoke the sympathies of Frederic

---

[1] Keats left England ravaged with Tuberculosis and headed on stormy seas towards Naples trying to write the finishing touches to his *"Bright Star"*. He was left in quarantine for 10 days before embarking in Rome certain that [he had] *"an habitual feeling of my real life having past, and that I am leading a posthumous existence."* [Last letter written by Keats to Charles Armitage Brown November 30th 1820]. Keats had moved into Brown's house after Keats' brother had died of Tuberculosis. After this Brown managed all of Keats' affairs and financial matters.

From a never completed book on Belgium by Charles Baudelaire. *Sur la Belgique, epilogue, Complete Works, vol. 2, ed. Yves-Gérard le Dantec, rev. by Claude Pichois (1976).*

© The Author(s), under exclusive license to Springer Nature Switzerland AG 2022   77
A. P. Zbar, *Syphilis*, https://doi.org/10.1007/978-3-031-08968-8_5

Chopin (1810–1849) abandoned in his terminal Tuberculosis by his lover Georges
Sand (1804–1876) who saw fit to recreate his allusion in her play *Lucrezia Floriani*
that portrayed him more as a whining infant than the most romantic notion of an
exhausted genius too ill to compose.[2]

So too there has been no book in the literature of syphilology quite like that of
Albert Camus' *The Plague* describing not only in detail the lymphatic spread and
putrefying death of those so afflicted but using the power of an epidemic as a
political allegory.[3] Undoubtedly, the carnal genesis of Syphilis (although potentially a great font of romantic notions), could somehow never transcend the coital
origins of the disease sufficiently so as to create its own iconic literature. Nor too
could its most pestilential features or the terminal ravings of its neurosphilitic
victims evoke either a sympathy of the reading classes or sufficient identification
with its protagonists so as to result in any sort of treasured literary canon.

That of course is not to say that less iconic or less well-known plays and novels do
not either centrally or peripherally address the issue or that Syphilis is not lightly
insinuated into our portrait galleries. Syphilis would litter the satires of Jonathan
Swift, Samuel Johnson and John Locke and the prose of Sir Thomas More, John
Donne and Erasmus, but the poets Dryden and Pope would steer well clear of the
subject. The drama of Syphilis would be portrayed by the Bavarian Oscar Panizza
(1853–1921) whose 1895 play *The Council of Love (Das Liebeskonzil): A Celestial
Tragedy* landed him a year in prison after its debut following conviction in Munich
on 93 separate counts of blasphemy. In it, Divine roles are characterized more than
anything for their distinctly human traits. So God is depicted as senile and indecisive,
Jesus as depressed and ineffectual and the Virgin Mary as a harlot with only Satan
himself appearing as a model of coordinated intellect conspiring to infect Mankind.
Here, Syphilis arrives in the form of the beguiling Salome.[4] Panizza dedicated the

---

[2] Chopin became so enfeebled by Tuberculosis that Sand who began devotedly to nurse him ended
up describing him as her "*third child*" and as a "*beloved little corpse*". After publication in 1847 of
her *Lucrezia Floriani*, the allusions in the play to Chopin proved so intolerable that the couple split
never to meet one another again. When Chopin's sister Ludwika transferred the raft of letters
between them back to Sand, it is thought that Sand burned them. Aspersions have been cast on the
more romantic end of Chopin's life wracked with Tuberculosis suggesting rather that he might
have suffered from a congenital pulmonary illness (either cystic fibrosis or the much rarer
alpha-1-anti-trypsin deficiency). Resolution of this question could be made by DNA sampling of
his exhumed heart (which is separately buried in Warsaw's Holy Cross Church away from his
main remains at Père Lachaise in Paris), but perhaps rather than spoiling a nostalgic image the
Polish Government has persistently declined to cooperate.

[3] *La Peste* by Albert Camus (1913–1960) describes the ramifications of a sweeping plague in the
Algerian city of Oran outlining in detail the clinical lymphatic buboes of the disease. Although
alluding to an outbreak of cholera in 1849 under French colonization it is seen by many as a
reflection on the Nazi occupation of France and the impact of the French resistance movement.

[4] In the final scene the Devil defines the natural outcome of unmitigated disease in a victim where
"*At the end of a year his nose will fall into his soup.....He will gasp for hope like a dessicated
carp....If he is a Protestant he will become a Catholic, and* vice versa." [*transl.* French as *Le
concile d'amour*. Reference from edition Jean-Jacques Pauvert (Libertes) 1964]. Panizza's play
served as the inspiration for the German expressionist painter George Grosz's *The Funeral*

play to the Renaissance chronicler of the first Syphilis epidemic in Europe Ulrich von Hutten who in 1519 remained unshaken in his belief that *"those entrusted with the Holy Scriptures said that the Pox was the result of Divine wrath"*.[5] Panizza's stint as a consultant psychiatrist in Munich's mental asylum between 1882 and 1884 might have only served him to identify with some of his patients and he succumbed to a paranoid delusional illness most likely the tertiary manifestations of advanced Syphilis which he admitted that he had contracted as a student.[6]

Syphilis (at least in some of the literature), had been confined to the corners of society inhabited by the languid poets and the playwrights each living in the dank and squalid periphery of a world primarily populated by prostitutes, vagrants and suffering artists. It had spawned the very model of the *poète maudit* (the accursed poet), marginalized from the wider world, drug- and absinthe-addled like the literary lovers Paul Verlaine and Arthur Rimbaud, each destined for the misguided impression of a romantically premature death.[7]

Before he had won the Nobel Prize for literature in 1907, Rudyard Kipling (1865–1936) had written his short story the *Love-o'-women* as part of a collection [the] *Many Inventions*. It was as he prefaced *"a lamentable tale of things, done long ago and ill done"* and was perhaps one of the first accurate descriptions of advanced neurosyphilis. It is the story of the hapless soldier (stationed in India and serving in

---

(executed in 1917) which depicted a funeral procession populated by what Grosz described as *"a hellish procession of dehumanized figures… reflecting alcohol, syphilis, plague…a protest against a humanity that had gone insane, …a gin alley of grotesque dead bodies and madmen…. a teeming throng of possessed human animals…[that] wherever you step, there's the smell of shit"*. It supposedly represented his frustration with German society emerging from World War 1 and was a vanguard of the *Neue Sachlichkeit* (New Objectivity) movement sweeping literature and art in Weimar Germany.

[5] From Ulrich van Hutten's *De guiaci medicina et morbo gallico*. (Mainz 1519 with German and French translations in 1520). Panizza's obsession with Catholicism almost certainly stemmed from his early childhood where he and his siblings were all baptized but following his father's death as a young child his mother had petitioned to bring the children up as Protestant. His plays demonstrated a militant distrust of what he regarded as Catholic hypocrisy and which he felt were exemplified under the papacy of Rodrigo Borgia (Alexander VI) in the 15th Century. See C. Quetel. *Ibid: 45*.

[6] Panizza's personal battles were recounted in his 1904 autobiography where he admits that although his Syphilis was treated that he was still suffering abscesses in his legs (most likely gummatous disease). Following a lecture that he gave entitled *"On Genius and Madness"* (*Genie und Wahnsinn*) he was publicly recognized to be delusional and was confined to the Herzogshöhe mental institution in Bayreuth for the last 16 years of his life. Judgments on his sanity were also influenced by a suicide attempt in 1904 and an arrest for indecent exposure protesting down the main streets of Munich wearing only a shirt. This event occurred after the local psychiatric institute had refused to examine and treat his mother.

[7] The term *poète maudit* was originally coined by Alfred de Vigny (1797–1863) in his 1832 novel *Stello* which examined the inherent conflict between the imaginations of the poet and the desire to represent basic societal truths. It has come to reflect the troubled poetic genius destined through physical abuse from drugs and alcohol (and perhaps even sexual overexcitement!) to suffer a premature death.

the Black Tyrone Regiment), Larry Tighe[8] whose legendary prowess as a womanizer had earned him the sobriquet, the *'Love-o'-women'*. For Kipling, Tighe could *"put the comether on any woman that trod the Green earth av God"*.[9] The small tale vividly recounts the latter life of Tighe suffering the traumas of repeated painful syphilitic tabetic crises.

By the time of writing. Kipling had just moved with his new wife Caroline Balestier to Vermont and had felt compelled to write the story at the same time as he was formulating his most famous works *The Jungle Book* and *Captains Courageous.* In it, Tighe appears, staggering and reeling in his gait and stamping his feet along the ground to hear them slap down as those do whose peripheral sensory nerves are so destroyed that they cannot feel the position of their feet as they walk. Kipling's military doctor Lowndes asks Tighe to stand still and straight with his eyes shut, *"not hould* [ing] *by your comrade;"* a literal description of a neurologic sign first described in 1840 by Moritz Romberg (1795–1873)[10] as a characteristic of any degenerative neurologic disorder affecting the sensory function of the limbs. Tighe confirms for him an inability to even perform this simple task. *"Tis all up …I'd fall doctor, an' you know ut"* he says accepting his own well-perceived limitations that he could neither feel his own feet or where they were in space.[11] Such was the general awareness of advanced Syphilis at the time that Tighe, sufficiently cognizant of his disorder, so suggested the diagnosis to his attending physician when his unsteadiness of gait

---

[8] Tighe's position as a "gentleman ranker" placed him as an enlisted man derived from the aristocratic class and would suggest some prior indiscretion. Tighe's recklessness under fire (which Kipling portrayed as almost suicidal) was most likely a feature of a sense of invincibility which would have been inflamed (so to speak) by underlying neurosyphilis and which would fit with the grandiose behaviours which are a terminal presentation of the illness.

[9] Larry (Kipling wrote) had been *"suckled by a she-devil"* and *"his face was like the face av a divil that has been cooked too long"*.

[10] Romberg noted the finding in those with a principally proprioceptive disorder (a sensory ataxia which causes someone to sway and teeter where they cannot determine without visual or auditory clues where their limbs are in spatial orientation). This feature can also be observed in those with inherent balance problems or visual disturbances so that it is not unique to neurosphyilis and as a simple examination it has of course remained a part of any sobriety test. Romberg particularly used it in his practice as a syphilitic marker describing the feelings of his patients' limbs as if *"they were covered in fur."* Tighe recognizes his limitations reporting that *"for a week an' more I was kickin' my toes against stones an' stumps for the pleasure av feelin' thim hurt"*.

[11] At the time tabes dorsalis was generally known to the public as "locomotor ataxia" (a term coined initially by Guillaume Duchenne in 1858). Kipling would have been aware of this association by his personal acquaintance with Sir William Gowers who reported the connection as a series of cases in the *Lancet* in 1881 and who was a personal friend and through his (i.e. Kipling's) association with William Osler (the Regius Professor of Medicine at Oxford) who had just published details of neurosyphilis in his *Principles and Practice of Medicine* (1892). Kipling in his story playfully suggests that locomotor ataxia was so called because it ran over its victims *"like a locomotive"*, rather than reflecting its impingement as a primary paralysing movement disorder. He was well aware of its venereal origins and significance when his protagonist Tighe admits that he acquired the disease from *"bein' called Love-o'-women"*.

became so obvious to others that it could no longer be hidden from view.[12] The story ends even more tragically, as if it had come from a Shakespearean playbook. Tighe ends his days in a brothel amazingly enough supported by his long-suffering wife, his *"Di'monds-an-Pearls"*.[13] Her shame is so great that she kills herself there with a pistol. All the doctor could do (arriving so drunk he is described as *"full as a tick"*) is attribute both deaths to *"most naturil causes"*[14] and unchastened by Kipling's moral lesson Lowndes runs away with a major's wife immediately after the funeral ceremony.

Although it may seem unfair to suggest, much of the literary legend of the *"morbo Gallico"* has been the chronicle of the lives of French novelists. Charles Baudelaire (1821–1867) and Gustave Flaubert (1821–1880) were admiring friends but also cousins in syphilitic suffering. Born in the same year, Flaubert outlived the more promiscuous Baudelaire who keeping his illness secret from the public, openly wrote of his syphilitic travails to friends and even respectfully to his mother.[15] Baudelaire's constant fretting about his health seemed justified. *"I believe that I am sick and a sick man even if the sickness is imagined is a sick man"*,[16] he wrote. Such a rant would have been music indeed to any hypochondriac's ears. But it is hard in his case to separate the symptomatology of an ailing neurosyphilitic from an underlying drug-addled antisocial whose reported episodes of extreme violence and even cruelty would have been spurred on intermittently by repeated exposure to a cocktail of laudanum, opium, belladonna, quinine and valerian. In there somewhere his fevers, lancinating abdominal pains, rheumatics and depression would all have fit with the diagnosis of Syphilis either in each of the individual symptoms masquerading as other complaints or as a whole. In the finish, he was sent paralysed and unable to speak first to the Sisters of Charity, (so appalled by his blasphemous hand gestures that they refused to take him) and thence to the aptly named converted asylum the Hôtel du Grand Miroir. For wrecks like this the favourite final common resting place was Dr. Esprit Blanche's asylum at Passy.

---

[12] Tighe in desperation cries *"Niver did I know that a man cud enjure such tormint widout his heart crackin' in his ribs"*. The doctor, aghast at the idea that Tighe might know of his condition retorts *"Holy Shmoke! "an' who are you to be givin' names to your diseases? Tis agin all the reg'lations"*.

[13] Confined to a hospital bed unable to walk, (calling himself *"a living carpse"*) Tighe sensing the end prefers to return to a local brothel and had sufficient power when he arrived to walk unaided up its front verandah steps.

[14] The regiment he felt *"will be thankful for wan grave the less to dig"*. So ends the story with the aphorism *"there are times,…whin tis better for the man to die than to live an' by consequince forty million time betther for the woman"*.

[15] Despite many supporting Baudelaire's censored writings (notably Flaubert and also Paul Verlaine), many considered not only his works but his lifestyle fairly debauched and reprehensible. Baudelaire's *Les Fleurs du Mal* had at its release been censored for obscenity by the French Public Safety Section of the Interior Ministry. Although his promiscuity was legendary, many also questioned his sexual orientation as well as his proclivity. André Gide thought that Baudelaire was a virgin and Marcel Proust was convinced that Baudelaire was homosexual.

[16] Hayden *Ibid* p. 116.

Flaubert watching from the sidelines had also experienced sustained speculation about his own love life (not restricting himself to one gender) even if he had been publicly more forthcoming about his syphilitic woes.[17] Found in his bath in Croisset after yet another seizure his colleague de Maupassant (1850–1893) noted with dismay a bruised and blackish collar mark around his neck (writing to his friend Turgenev about it in the way authors do to sensationalize one anothers' death). It had led to speculation that Flaubert in despair over his illness had taken his own life. For Guy de Maupassant, there was much greater openness to his own fight with Syphilis if only he could link its acquisition to his heightened sexual prowess. Syphilis was worn as a badge of honour and it was part and parcel of the professed sexual proclivity of a man who claimed to be multi-orgasmic and to suffer no refractory ejaculatory periods between encounters. De Maupassant in his boasting rhetoric comes across as an absolute rake proudly and busily infecting as many prostitutes as he could find and even at one stage crudely daubing the image of a small chancre on his penis and forcing himself on one woman after first showing her its horror.

It was a reverse threat to their congress, he with a more ultimate and defining power of their union than almost any counter-infection she could bestow. His would never be a life of remorse writing in frenzy of the unromantic notions of the recriminations inflicted by unremitting advanced syphilitic illness in his pathetic story *Bed Number 29* (Le Lit 29). It tells of the handsome Captain Epivent travelling to the Franco-Prussian War after one night of passionate love with the young beauty Irma only to return after battle to find her emaciated, confused and dying in a Syphilis ward.[18] As with others, de Maupassant's end was ignominious wandering the streets of Paris, violently shouting, confabulating and raving with delusions of grandeur. In the finish, he would claim to have planted small trees which would grow up into tiny versions of himself and he was found licking the walls of his asylum cell wrapped in a straight-jacket. When released from its constraints he spent his time spilling over his urinal bottles in the search for hidden jewels.

France too would cradle in death Oscar Wilde (1854–1900), a man so disappointed with life that he could only summon up the energy in the finish to pick a fight with his drab wallpaper.[19] Even his terminal embrace of the Catholic faith (albeit for a short while) would not save him and he died in the Hotel d'Alsace in Paris in abject poverty having suffered the humiliation of witnessing the wholesale auctioning off of his most precious library. Before then he had portentously

---

[17] Flaubert had confessed in a letter in 1849 that he had contracted the disease as a young man whilst travelling through Egypt, writing to his friend Louis Bouilhet (1821–1869) of the need to bandage his penis to cover slowly weeping chancres so that he could ride a horse from Marmaris to Smyrna. [See Francis Steigmuller Ed Tr. *The Letters of Gustave Flaubert 1830–1857*. Cambridge Harvard University Press 1980: 117]. Whilst in Cairo, Flaubert had visited hospital wards to look at the young men openly displaying their anal chancres to the public.

[18] *Complete Short Stories of Guy de Maupassant*. New York Doubleday 1955.

[19] Wilde was reputed to have said on his deathbed *"My wallpaper and I are fighting a duel to the death. One or other of us has got to go"*.

predicted his descent into madness that he felt sure followed the inadequate drainage of a chronic middle ear infection.[20] Syphilis as a cause of this complaint was only considered by Arthur Ransome (1884–1967) in a biography where he at least waited with some decorum a dozen years after Wilde's death to even suggest the diagnosis.[21] Wilde's acolyte and benevolent biographer Robert Sherard (1861–1943) had tried desperately to deflect attention from Wilde's homosexual proclivities (advanced by André Gide) by suggesting that Wilde had acquired Syphilis as a young man from a campus whore called *"Old Jess"* who roamed Oxford's Magdalen College. As a strategy to rehabilitate Wilde with a heterosexual patina it proved singularly unsuccessful.[22]

Wilde having stood accused and convicted of having performed indecencies with Lord Alfred 'Bosie' Douglas (1870–1945) did not live long enough to see Bosie's denial of his own homosexuality and the libel trials which came to dominate Bosie's life. Like Wilde, Douglas had embraced the Catholic faith and married. Perhaps as cover he became an ardent critic of London's homosexual enclaves describing Wilde in the homophobic journal *Vigilante* as *"the greatest force for evil that has appeared in Europe during the last three hundred and fifty years"*.[23]

---

[20] The infection most likely commenced whilst Wilde was in prison but there is considerable debate concerning its aetiology. Some have suggested that it was a common, garden variety infection that had spread to his mastoid sinuses and which when inadequately treated progressed to a delayed brain infection. Others have suggested that it was a specific tumour of the middle ear (called a cholesteatoma) which was also inadequately treated. The possibility that it represented an advanced stage of neurosyphilis (which may or may not have been secondarily infected with other bacteria) has been proffered by many separate sources.

[21] Ransome Arthur. *Oscar Wilde: A Critical Study*. Mitchell Kennerley New York 1912. Dedicated to Robert Ross.

[22] Robert Sherard. *Oscar Wilde: The Story of an Unhappy Friendship*. London Hermes Press 1902. Sherard's beguiling obsession with Wilde reinforced the benign nature of Wilde's illnesses in *The Life of Oscar Wilde* (T. Werner Laurie1906) and *The Real Oscar Wilde* (T Werner Laurie 1917). Sherard's own credentials could not have been more impeccable. He was William Wordsworth's great grandson and became entranced by Wilde at the height of his powers when they met at the Hôtel Voltaire. Gide was much more likely to be believed since he participated with Wilde in homosexual encounters, naming a young 'rent-boy' whom he called Mohammed and whom he had witnessed Wilde picking up in Algiers. It had been rumoured that '*Old Jess*' had also infected Lord Randolph Churchill, Winston Churchill's father.

[23] Even though Douglas lost a different libel suit against Ransome, the offending pages concerning Douglas' relationship with Wilde were removed in subsequent editions. By some irony, Winston Churchill successfully sued Lord Alfred Douglas for libel in 1923 with Douglas spending 6 months in London's Wormwood Scrubs prison after asserting that Churchill would privately benefit from the release of false information concerning the outcome of the Battle of Jutland in World War 1. Worse still Douglas had anti-semitically reported that it had all been to enhance a group of Jewish financiers once British stocks expectedly fell in value after the false announcement. Whilst in prison in 1924 Douglas paid homage to Wilde's *De Profundis* (From the Depths) by writing his own poetic work *In Excelsis* (From the Heights). Although there were established camps to comment on Wilde's sexual proclivities, Sherard's attempts to rehabilitate Wilde by claiming that all his *"mental, moral and physical aberrations"* stemmed from an unfortunate legacy of indiscreet heterosexual sex (and worse as some bravado that he deliberately infected others) came to nought. Others too tried to provide some heterosexual narrative for Wilde pointing

For Wilde, much of the external impression of his life was bravado and obfuscation, attributing the terminal blotches covering most of his skin to be the result of eating bad mussels (rather than the effect of cutaneous syphilides). In magnanimity, he did at least acknowledge that his drinking of over a litre of brandy a day might have also contributed to his poor state of health.[24] Syphilis or no, Wilde's profligacy and arrogance reflected an underestimate of those enemies who had mobilized against him and his fall from grace was as much an act of self-destruction as any external humiliation. Perhaps its effects on his brain had weakened his sense of self-preservation and the radar that warns of personal danger over fanciful paranoia. If Syphilis was running its course in Wilde as he languished in penury at the Hôtel d'Alsace, it would be just another addition to his internal conflict and perhaps like other great artistic figures, just another secret.[25]

The physical legacy of its procurement would occupy the French satirist Voltaire who wrote in his *Candide ou L'optimisme* and in his *L'homme aux quarante écus* of the line of procession as it passes from one victim to the next heeding neither the boundaries of social class nor their personal stature.[26] The movement of infection reads like the Biblical succession of begatting in Genesis[27] where *"Paquette [that pretty wench who waited on our noble Baroness] had this present from a very learned Franciscan Grey Friar... he had had it of an old Countess, who had received it from a cavalry Captain, who owed it to a Marchioness, who took it from a page, who had received it from a Jesuit.. who had it in a direct line from one of*

---

as evidence to his long-suffering wife Constance and to his two boys Cyril and Vyvyan. The 'heterosexual' story was also put about by his friend the poet Ernest Dowson (1867–1900) who claimed that upon Wilde's release from prison in 1897, that Dowson took Wilde almost immediately to a London brothel.

[24] His drinking was reported by the proprietor of the Hotel d'Alsace, Jules Dupoirier.

[25] Other notable authors rumoured to have suffered at some stage during their lives from Syphilis include James Joyce (1882–1941), Isak Dinesen (Karen Blixen—1885–1962), Lev Tolstoy, (1828–1910) and Heinrich Heine (1797–1856). Composers reputed to have Syphilis included Ludwig van Beethoven (1770–1827), Franz Schubert (1797–1828), Robert Schumann (1810–1856), Hugo Wolf (1860–1903), Bedrich Smetana (1824–1884) and Frederick Delius (1862–1934). In the case of Beethoven whose body was exhumed in 1862, samples of his inner ear and temporal bone proved inconclusive and did not advance the cause of death beyond what was written on his death certificate of *"Wassersucht"* (dropsy). In Schumann's case, his wife Clara admitted him to the Endenich asylum after Schumann's orchestral conducting became so difficult that he was forced to tie the baton onto his wrist with string (and perhaps so that she could carry on an affair with Johannes Brahms). Most of the debate in Schumann's case concerns other distinct psychiatric illnesses as differential diagnoses for Syphilis including manic depressive psychosis, schizophrenia, paranoia and obsessive compulsive disorder. Schubert was exhumed along with Beethoven and both heads were removed for Syphilis analysis (now both lost). As testament to the possibility that both had the disease, Schubert's and Beethoven's doctor Josef von Vering had written extensively on the management of the syphilitic in a book *Concerning the Treatment of Syphilis by Applying a Mercuric Liniment*.

[26] Voltaire née Francois-Marie Arouet (1694–1778) wrote *Candide* in 1759 and *L'homme aux quarante écus* in 1768.

[27] Genesis 5: 2–32.

the companions of Christopher Columbus".[28] Voltaire's line of succession leaves no doubt as to the origins of the European scourge and traces its contacts much as those suffering the first throes of HIV-AIDS were forced to chronicle and surrender the names of their lovers even when so many might have been anonymous. For others like the novelist Paul Vérola (1863–1931) in his 1891 Parisian novel *L'infamant* (The Infamous), Syphilis staked out its territory of attack and embarrassment only by class. "*Phthisis [TB] and typhoid fever are noble and aristocratic, apoplexy belongs to the rich bourgeoisie... the whole string of shameful diseases that no one admits to or acknowledges, epilepsy and syphilis turn any human being they enslave into a pariah*".

The literature would fall to one side or the other, either in shame or in defiant pride at each rendition of the news of the arrival of Syphilis on to a new victim and at a time when its transition was a death sentence. Théophile Gautier (1811–1872) in his *Lettres à la Présidente* recording his travels through Italy rejoiced in the unadulterated splendid and very public nature of the expressions of the Pox "*as pure as the time of Francis I*" revelling in its overt Renaissance symbolism. "*Boils are exploding in groins like shells, and purulent jets of clap vie with the fountains in the Piazza Navona*"[29] he wrote even if he like many had confused the ubiquity of gonorrhoea with the more occult presentations of Syphilis. For those enjoying Bernini's Fountain of the Four Rivers (his *Fontana dei Quattro Fiumi*) in Rome's famous piazza, the spewing streams could not be more symbolic and each time I go there now, I think of Gautier and always feel a tiny sense of shame.

Only the unique manner in which it would attack the visceral systems of the body could be its distinguishing mark. For Michel Corday (1869–1937) whose military career had spawned his novels on the barrack lives of his fellow soldiers, his *Venus* (*Venus ou Les Deux Risques*) of 1901 spoke of its imperiousness as an illness and of its selective destructive powers. The puppet Master to an almost innocent and unsuspecting marionette. "*It is a disease that chooses the part of its victim that is most appealing*" he wrote "*....suppressing the senses... it plays with a man as if he were a puppet ...making him jump and start...and then it tires of this Punchinello*" only to finally strike after all this spasmodic parody by rendering his limbs useless, flailing and ataxic. Beginning with twitching hyperactivity, it collapses and exhausts itself into a paralysis.

Somewhere, however, locked in its infection was the curiously reported ability that the *Treponeme* might possess in some so fortunate to actually enhance their genius. Rather than parading its destructive force amongst the cerebral detritus, it could stimulate others more susceptible to greatness. Who is to know if Friedrich Nietzsche's (1844–1900) spiralling descent into mental collapse was spurred on by a small bacillus and even as some have suggested in the works of de Maupassant or the prolific imagery

---

[28] *Candide* Chap. 4. *How Candide found his old Master Pangloss and what had happened to them.*

[29] See Quétel. *Ibid.* p. 294. *Secret Museum of the King of Naples,* Paris, 1890.

of Van Gogh, powered and sustained by the bacterium.[30] Syphilis, an essential requirement to genius! Even Nietzsche could stand aside from his lunacy and write his *Wahnzettel* ("Madness Letters") to Franz Liszt's daughter Cosima (1837–1930) and to his old Professor of History at Basle, Jacob Burkhardt (1818–1897). Passing through the doors of the Jena Clinic with his complex terminal madness Nietzsche was still sane enough to ensure the release of his book the *Twilight of the Idols.*

One may speculate like this on the workings of the brain and the chance for it to be positively exploited by a tiny bacterium and perhaps in the worst of circumstances equally postulate a capacity it might possess to corrupt. It was a morbid fear of the novelist Léon Daudet (1867–1942) that his father Alphonse (1840–1897) who had suffered from tertiary Syphilis had passed the germ on and made Léon himself a '*heredo*'. Both Daudets would be consumed by their visceral anti-Semitism, a hatred which in the father became more vociferous as his disease progressed and in the son too as he matured. The elder Daudet chronicles every painful twitch of his disabling *Tabes* in the slim volume *In The Land of Pain* (faithfully translated by Julian Barnes[31]) and finally reports how he was dominated by the imperative of pain which orbited that obsession. In the finish, the only living part of him became his relentless pain. The son, Léon proved himself to be even more on the wrong side of history and notoriously more rabid in his anti-Semitism than his father siding with the anti-Dreyfusards who had dominated the anti-semitic political agenda of France at the *fin de siècle*. Drawn to medicine to explain his familial ills, Léon abandoned his medical studies on the cusp of his final examinations and wrote one of his defining novels *Devant la douleur* drawing together a dystopian world populated by hereditary syphilitics, (he imagines) just like him. For Daudet, society's citizens were defined by a new syphilitic census which could only count as its registered members its "*neurasthenics...melancholics,.... misanthropists, maniaques and misfits*".[32]

---

[30] It is claimed by his biographer, Robert Sherard of de Maupassant that in the throes of advanced Syphilis, he was able to enter into the most productive period of his life, producing 300 short stories, 6 novels, 3 plays and a raft of poetry. [See Robert H. Sheridan. *The Life, Work and Evil Fate of Guy de Maupassant.* New York Brentano's 1926: p. 235]. de Maupassant and Theo and Vincent van Gogh were all at one time under the care of one of Paris' most committed syphilologists, David Gruby (who also looked after Alphonse Daudet, Heinrich Heine and Georges Sand). Of poor de Maupassant already mad his options for treatment were limited by his intense dislike of all things German including Professor Ehrlich's recent wonder drug Salvarsan.

[31] *In the Land of Pain*. Alphonse Daudet. Edited and translated by Julian Barnes New York: Alfred A. Knopf, 2002. In the book, Daudet narrates his bizarre treatments at one stage being suspended upside down by his jaw and injected with experimental remedies developed in Guinea pigs. Daudet was close friends with Edouard Drumont, (1844–1917) the founder of the Anti-Semitic League of France and the editor of the anti-Semitic newspaper *La Libre Parole* which ran from 1892 until 1924. Daudet, a leading anti-Dreyfusard, was a strong opponent of Dreyfus' supporters (the Dreyfusards) like Émile Zola, Georges Clemenceau, Sara Bernhardt and Anatole France who sided with Captain Alfred Dreyfus (1859–1935) against fraudulent assertions of his treason to the German embassy. Daudet was one of the staunchest advocates of the collaborationist Vichy régime and was also violently opposed to the Jewish reformer, Léon Blum (1872–1950) who was Prime Minister of France three times.

[32] Leon Daudet. *Devant la douleur.* 1915 Edn p. 172.

Speculating on the spirochaete's predilection to galvanize some impression of genius from a morass of ethnic hatred, he perhaps singles out some value in his father's mixed legacy. *"The microbe of this terrible disease, the treponema, since we must call it by its name"*, he writes, *"is as much the power behind genius and talent, heroism and wit as that behind general paralysis, tabes and almost all forms of degenerescence....it is the spirit, invisible but present which moves the romantic and the madcap, the sublime-looking misfit, the pedantic or the violent revolutionary."* For Daudet, it was the levelling that any hereditary ailment might arbitrarily produce to leave its mark on even the most ordinary of men making *"a great poet of a maid's son,... a satyr of a peaceful bourgeois."*[33]

The novelist Karen Blixen (1885–1962) too had recognized it, watching it starve her physical body so that in the end she looked like an emaciated bird. She was convinced that without the influence of Syphilis she would have never been able to write her great masterpieces, the *Seven Gothic Tales, Out of Africa* and the *Winter Tales*. In one story, her *Third Cardinal's Tale*, the dreaded disease is caught from the most devout of acts, kissing the foot of the statue of the apostle Peter in the Vatican after unbeknownst it had been contaminated by an ordinary Roman worker. In one simple act, it had democratized the transfer of Syphilis from the carnal aristocracy to the pious and then to the plebeian and it had sanitized their collective misfortune.[34]

For others, it would be pure paranoia that would signal their end and Syphilis' last fatal influence. Observing de Maupassant wandering the streets of Rouen during the unveiling of a statue in honour of Flaubert, his friend the literary critic Edmond de Goncourt (1822–1896) could not help himself. "[He is] *shrivelled up with pain, those big eyes at bay ...a protestation against an iniquitous fatality lit up with dying lights*" he wrote in paradox. This from a man whose brain served as a syphilitic background and who had once boasted of his ability to write an entire

---

[33] Daudet L. *Les Morticoles*. 1894. [See also Mary Donaldson-Evans. *Medical examinations: Dissecting the doctor in French narrative prose. 1857–1894*. Lincoln University of Nebraska 2000].

[34] Isak Dinesen (Blixen K). T*he Third Cardinal's Tale* in *Last Tales*. New York Vintage 1957; 97–8. In this simple gesture she speaks of the protagonist (and virgin) Lady Flora Gordon lingering at the kiss to smell the *"smell of sweat and the stable,... a smell of the people"* and to contract Syphilis through no fault of her own (as Blixen believed of herself). The book was initially rejected by the English Book Society and by the Book of the Month Club even as Blixen was writing it as she described with *"a foot and a half in the grave"*.

short story in one sitting without a single correction.[35] Tortured by lancinating ocular pain and headaches, incoherent and paretic, de Maupassant still had time for his libidinous orgies. But was it de Maupassant himself who had challenged the syphilitic organism or was it the other way around with Syphilis weakening his moral fibre?

By contrast, the allusions to Syphilis in painting are somewhat obtuse but if anything they are exemplified more in the face of one man, Gerard de Lairesse (1641–1711) rather than in any allegory. De Lairesse, the son of the painter Renier (1597–1667) quickly developed a local fame training with Rembrandt and dividing his time between Cologne and Aix-la-Chapelle particularly following his indiscretions that necessitated sudden departure from his home town of Liège.[36, 37] De Lairesse painted two self-portraits, one now in the Musèe Bonnat in France's Ville de Bayonne and the other of a more sedate and less troubled man held in the Uffizi Gallery in Florence. The second image although seemingly more confident, clearly acknowledges his own facial shortcomings which would have been familiar to anyone exposed to the chidhood facies of Europe's *hérédos*. There he boldly shows his saddle nose with its collapsed bridge and its tip rolled up,[38] the chin jutting, the lips overly full and the bossed prominent brows that would beyond the time of Lairesse ultimately be well described by the French paediatrician Jules Parrot (1829–1883).

It didn't stop de Lairesse in his ambitions and he dabbled in his great love, the theatre, as a set designer until his eyesight failed so badly that he was confined to his home. Realizing that his congenital Syphilis would eventually destroy him, he became one of Europe's premier art critics writing his influential *Groot Schilderboek* (The Book of Great Painters) in 1707 and tutoring on the theoretical

---

[35] See *f.n. 30*. [Sherard, Robert. *The Life, Work and Evil Fate of Guy de Maupassant*. New York Brentanos, *Ibid.* p. 360.]. Even this accomplishment scored for de Maupassant the sexual nature of any conquest. "*It was there*" he wrote of the story "*complete, erect, within my mind*". [Quoted in Hayden, Deborah. Basic Books 2003. *Ibid.* pp. 149]. See also Georges Normandy. *La Fin de Maupassant*. 1927 Paris and Jean Lacassagne. *Guy de Maupassant et son mal*. 1951.

[36] Legend has it that he was forced from his home after he was discovered to have been sleeping with two sisters who were modelling for him.

[37] The book was inspired by similar critiques by two artists turned art theorists, Karel van Mander's (1548–1606) *Schilder-Boeck* of 1604 on Netherlandish painting and Samuel Dirksch van Hoogstraten's (1627–1678) *Introduction to the Academy of Painting, or the Visible World* (the *Inleyding tot de hooge schoole der schilderkonst: anders de zichtbaere werelt*) of 1678. De Lairesse was highly regarded by Houbracken whom he included in his list of the greatest painters, the *De groote schouburgh der Nederlantsche konstschilders en schilderessen* of 1718.

[38] *Le pointe du nez retrousse* (the tip of the nose is rolled up).

aspects of painting. It was a major comedown for someone who was Rembrandt's natural successor in an era whose mercantile class revelled in de Lairesse's ornate Baroque style of the group portraiture of the Netherlands' wealthy guildmasters and burghers.[39] By all accounts Rembrandt loved him like his own[40] and yet felt compelled to paint him with a raw realism which acknowledged the illness over which Gerard had no control. It is almost like a photographic testament to the genetic imprint of a disease which had yet to be described but which on reading the accounts of the small children grown with advanced Syphilis 200 years later, can be visually checked off against Rembrandt's 17th Century portrait.[41] In stark contrast to Rembrandt's dark colours so much a feature of the sketchier style that marked his late phase, sits the young de Lairesse with the drawn pallor of a sickly man no one would particularly want to spend time around. As if in confirmation the art critic Arnold Houbraken (1660–1719) had written that colleagues first catching sight of de Lairesse "*gazed at him in horror because of his nauseating appearance*".[42] Other etchings with dubious attribution now in the British Museum clearly show the same unusual facial features so evident to Rembrandt.

If he did have congenital Syphilis, it did not (like some) slow him down intellectually and he was regarded with great respect as clever and personable if not lascivious and above all, possessed of a magnetic charm for the ladies. His love of theatre drew him to the surgeon-anatomist and erstwhile playwright Govaert Bidloo (1649–1713) whose magnum opus on human dissection the *Anatomia Humani Corporis* de Lairesse illustrated in 1685.[43] The idea of one of the grimy anatomists seeking out a prominent artist to accurately redraw their dissections of cadavers as they occurred in real time was not new having been introduced by the Belgian anatomist Andreas Vesalius (1514–1564) who had commissioned the painter Jan Stefan van Calkar (1499–1546) a student of the great Venetian Master, Titian to execute all of the anatomical dissection drawings in his 1543 textbook the *Fabrica de*

---

[39] His French style of painting was compared to that of Nicolas Poussin and de Lairesse was often referred to as the "Dutch Poussin".

[40] Rembrandt's first son Rumbartus died in infancy in 1635 as did his daughter Cornelia in 1638. His only other legitimate son Titus (1641–1668) with whom he was exceptionally close died from the plague one year before a heartbroken Rembrandt himself died (1606–1669).

[41] The appearances of children suffering from congenital Syphilis were first reported by Sir Jonathan Hutchinson in 1858 in a paper he read to the British Medical Association entitled: "*On the means of recognizing the subjects of inherited syphilis in adult life*". The link between congenital Syphilis and Rembrandt's portrait of de Lairesse was made in 1913 by Dr. J.H. Hanken as suggested first in an article by the Rijksmuseum director Frederik Schmidt-Degener (1881–1941).

[42] See Horton A. Johnson. *Gerard de Lairesse: Genius among the Treponemes. Journal of the Royal Society of Medicine.* 2004; Vol. 97: pp. 301–3.

[43] G. Bidloo printed in Dutch as *Ontleding des Menschelijken Lichaams* (*Dissection of the Human Body*) 1689.

humani corporis (On the Fabric of the Human Body).[44] De Lairesse's approach in the Bidloo book to display all of the layers of dissection showing the relationship of the muscles, tendons and sinews to one another in three dimensions was unique and both books by Vesalius and Bidloo came to dominate anatomical teaching in Europe following their publication, in no short measure due to the artwork involved.

Perhaps the fiery temperament of both men ultimately pushed them apart. Bidloo had a reputation for subterfuge and plagiarism in his work and was irascible and a known schemer in his dealings with fellow surgeons in Amsterdam's Guild. It had forced him to move to Leiden where he was appointed Rector and he moved even further afield as King Willem's personal physician after the Monarch was crowned King William III of England, Scotland and Northern Ireland.[45] de Lairesse was a particularly harsh critic of his own Master at one stage referring to Rembrandt's late period paintings as "*like muck running down the canvas (gelyk drek).*" But de Lairesse still imposed Bidloo's imagery with a distinct humanity that he had inherited from other Dutch painters of the Golden Age. Despite his conformity, de Lairesse still regarded Rembrandt's images of the Dutch peasantry as unworthy of the loftiest ambitions of art which should (he felt) be to uplift the human race. The images he made for Bidloo's cadavers were always discreetly dressed in their nightclothes even when the rest was splayed open in an impersonal manner. The identity of the corpse was always preserved and protected.[46]

---

[44] Vesalius' approach revolutionized the conduct of cadaver dissection in the anatomy schools across Europe and van Calkar's imagery dominated anatomic teaching manuals for the next 300 years. Although there is some debate concerning the artist in Vesalius' *De Fabrica humani corporis*, the Italian chronicler of Renaissance art, Giorgio Vasari (1511–1574) clearly attributes these images to him in his *Lives of the Most Excellent Painters, Sculptors, and Architects* 1550. The Oxford anatomist Thomas Willis (1621–1675) had by example used Sir Christopher Wren (1632–1723) as the artist sitting by his dissections of the human brain for Willis's 1664 *Cerebri anatome: cui accessit nervorum descriptio et usus.* Although Bidloo had himself been accused of plagiarism, he was also subject to rank copying. The English surgeon William Cowper (1666–1709) who most likely purchased engraved plates of de Lairesse's illustrations, then went on to republish them under his own name as *The Anatomy of the Humane Bodies* in 1698 in Latin without acknowledgement either to Bidloo or de Lairesse. This issue is examined in detail in Paule Dumaître's *La curieuse destinée des planches anatomiques de Gérard de Lairesse peintre en Hollande. Lairesse, Bidloo, Cowper* (Nieue Nederlandse Bijdragen, tot de Geschiedenis der Geneeskunde en der Natuurwetenschappen, no 6) Amsterdam Rodopi 1982.

[45] William, Prince of Orange was Statdholder of Holland, Zeeland, Utrecht, Gelderland and Overijssel and became King of England in 1689. Bidloo became his personal physician in 1695. Bidloo's son Nicolaas (1673/4–1735) was the personal physician to Tsar Peter the Great and established Moscow's first medical school.

[46] The original drawings of de Lairesse remain in the Réserve de la Bibliothèque de la Faculté de Médecine de Paris and according to the Wellcome Foundation librarian William Schupbach were purchased after de Lairesse's death by the physician Théodore Tronchin (1709–1781).

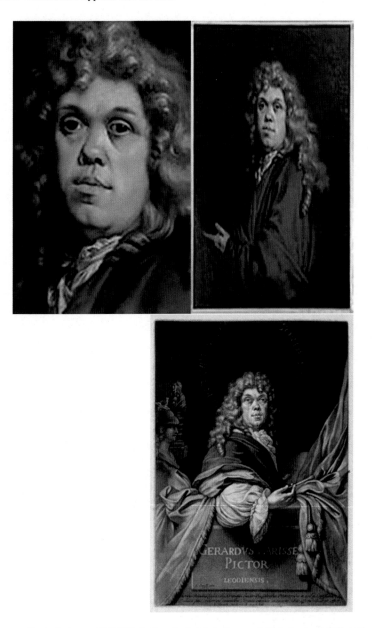

Top images: G. de Lairesse (? 1699) Self-portrait (plus close-up) Galeria degli Uffizi Florence.
Lower image: Portrait of Gerard de Lairesse British Museum Attributed to Pieter Schenk the Elder
(1660–1711) 1877,0210.169

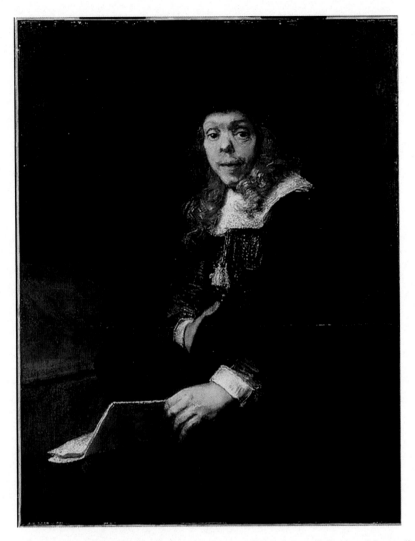

Rembrandt van Rijn. Portrait of Gerard de Lairesse 1665. Lehman Collection. Metropolitan Museum of Art. New York

Bidloo, perhaps more interested in the libretti of farces and satires that he wrote, (now appointed the Director of the Amsterdam theatre), frequently clashed with de Lairesse over the style of the images with de Lairesse trading anatomical accuracy for artistic license. In one famous drawing of an abdominal dissection there is an errant housefly crawling across part of a rotting carcass. The impudent realism of de Lairesse and perhaps his connection to the artistic establishment no matter how tenuous proved simply too much for Bidloo and far more than either man had bargained for. Anatomist and artist parted professional company never to work together again.

Leaving de Lairesse, the images of Syphilis are sparse and somewhat uncertain. There is Hans Holbein the Younger's *Head of a Young Man* covered along his face and neck with pustules which of course may or may not be the ravages of secondary Syphilis as much as a case of leprosy or the simple infectious blisters of childhood impetigo. The image was reputed to have penciled on its back "*Portrait of Ulrich van Hutten*" and it is emblazoned at the top with the mark 1523, the exact year of von Hutten's premature death.[47] The satirical artist and caricaturist William Hogarth (1697–1764) too, a man driven by a moral imperative and notoriously puritanical would often paint judgmental pieces that warned of Divine retribution on an unrepentant life. In his *Marriage à-la-mode* painted between 1743 and 1745, the third of his images of a newly married couple, *The Inspection,* clearly shows the now syphilitic and unfaithful Viscount, Lord Squanderfield with the blackened blotched marks on his neck typical of advancing Syphilis visiting an equally syphilitic doctor perhaps based upon Dr Richard Rock who had already appeared in Hogarth's *Harlots Progress*.[48] It is something more than a consultation and the aristocrat communes, smiling with the doctor in the presence of a woman, (perhaps a local brothel Madam herself covered in abstemes and furuncles) as if his disorder is merely an irritant of the most inconsequential nature. Here there was always complex allegory. Some images would be of unchaste women rising in boudoirs that reeked off the canvas with the effort of raucous lovemaking. The *beau désordre* of their rooms would be populated by cats (signifying sexual receptiveness) warily eyeing birds in flight (symbols of the male genitalia). The story of Squanderfield is a syphilitic mirror and takes on the mantle of a playwright's tragedy. In the finish he is killed by his wife's lover before Syphilis can take him. The lover is then executed and the Viscountess commits suicide.

---

[47] Tantalizingly, the pencilled-in inscription became erased somewhere between 1876 and 1910.

[48] In the 18th Century venereal disease was often referred to as the 'Alamode' disease, hence Hogarth's *Marriage-à-la-mode*. Dr Richard Rock was considered one of London's more notable quacks. [See Robert LS Cowley. *Marriage à la Mode: a Review of Hogarth's Narrative Art.* Manchester. Manchester University Press. 1983 and NF Lowe. Ch 10. *The Meaning of Venereal Diseases in Hogarth's Graphic Art.* In The Secret Malady (Ed). Linda E Merians *Ibid*: pp. 168–182].

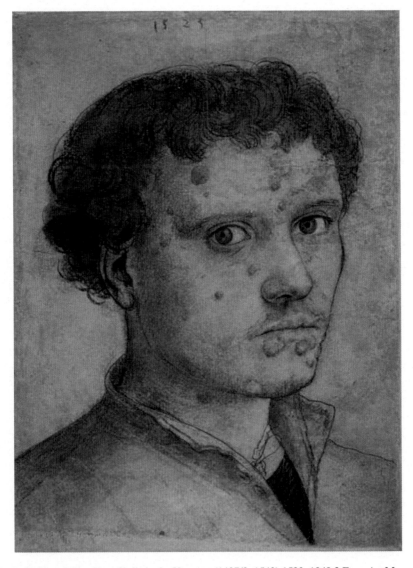

Head of a Young Man Hans Holbein the Younger (1497/8–1543) 1523. 1949.2 Fogg Art Museum
Cambridge Massachussetts USA Harvard Art Museums/Bequest of Paul J. Sachs Black ink and
red and yellow chalk

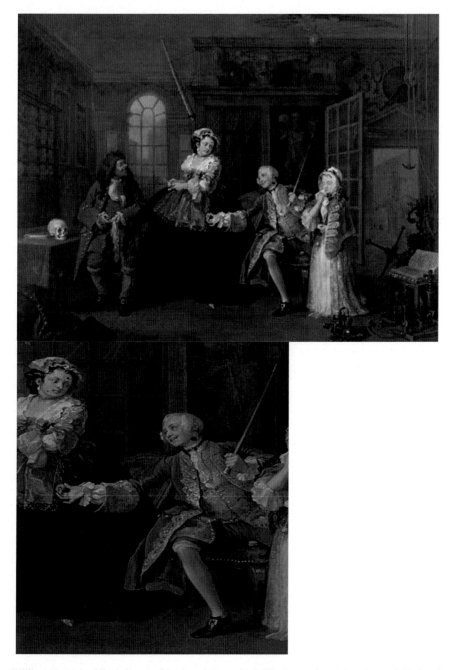

William Hogarth. Oil on Canvas. Marriage à-la-mode. 3. The Inspection. (plus close-up) National Gallery London

If Hogarth would have a natural successor, (at least in the artistic sense), it might have been Thomas Rowlandson (1756–1827). But that is where the comparison ends since Rowlandson through penury resorted for much of his life to the production of the sort of explicit erotic print that one might seek in the darkest Soho alleyways.[49] Rowlandson had particularly stiff competition for the pole position of London's premier caricaturist in the form of James Gillray (1757–1815) until Gillray's eyesight failed so badly that he felt compelled to throw himself out of a St. James Street window in an unsuccessful suicide attempt. Both Rowlandson and Gillray were expert at lampooning political figures across both sides of the channel in the wake of the French revolution and the Napoleonic Wars, with Gillray producing an amazing print of exhausted Pox-ridden French generals repatriated from the Battle of the Nile after a defeat at the hands of Lord Nelson in the earliest days of August 1798.[50] The scene is grim. In it, the unidentified officers report in exhaustion to a physician Lepaux most likely a parody of Dominique Larrey (1767–1842) Napoleon's Chief Surgeon of his Grand Armée. Lepaux (or Larrey) is holding up a urinal bottle with a copy of the "*Mal de Naples*" open on a desk crammed with specimens and diagnostic paraphernalia. To the left is a depleted bottle with the label Lake's Pills, (referring to Dr. Leake's pills), the most popular anti-Syphilis medication at the time. And further, standing upright two sarcophagi, one emblazoned with the word *Buonaparte* and the other that of his commander of the French forces in Egypt, Jean-Baptiste Kléber (recently assassinated by a disgruntled Syrian student). Below, one elderly emaciated French General is throwing up into a spittoon labelled simply *Jourdan*, the name of one of Napoleon's most loyal Marshals. The message was clear. Syphilis had infiltrated the very marrow of the French army, even right down to Larrey's sabre-like shinbones. For Rowlandson, by contrast, the true nature of the root of all evil was neither the Generals nor the Emperor himself, but rather women in general. Rowlandson would point his satiric finger in his *Six Stages of Mending a Face* where the decrepit could be covered by wigs and make-up. Their subterfuge could be detected in all its guile, if only someone like himself would simply expose their wily ways.

By 1901, Fournier had established the sternly named French Society of Sanitary and Moral Prophylaxis (*Societé Française de Prophylaxie Sanitaire et Morale*) as part of his drive to control the epidemic spread of the disease.[51] In amongst his prescriptions for the National illness were the mandated examinations and treatment of France's prostitutes, the source it was believed of the contagion those women and coquettish girls who still remained unregistered. Fournier was keen to draw together all the disparate arms of the National anti-Syphilis movement but more than this to solidify his place as a distinguished physician who was openly treating the real scourge of the time. Along the way he would modify the moral attitudes of society to suit his overarching views on how best to contain the disease.

---

[49] [See Oppe AP. *Thomas Rowlandson: his drawings and watercolours.* London The Studio Ltd 1923 and also Smith WG. T*he Amorous Illustrations of Thomas Rowlandson.* London Bibliophile Books 1983].

[50] The defeated French admiral Francois-Paul Brueys d'Aigalliers (1753–1798) was killed in the attack.

[51] Fournier had decided on the idea following the First International Syphilis Congress in 1899 which specifically examined Syphilis prevention.

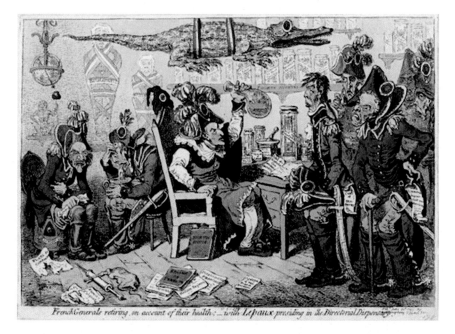

James Gillray. French Generals retiring on account of their health with Lepaux presiding in the Directorial Dispensary. Syphilis caricature with watercolours. 1799. British Library collection (with permission)

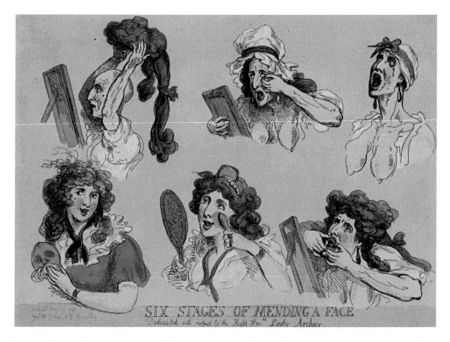

Thomas Rowlandson Six Stages of Mending a Face. 1792 Dedicated to Lady Sarah Archer (1741–1801). In some a wig, another covering her lifeless eyes, dentures for her toothless mouth and rouging her pallor to make herself presentable. Metropolitan Museum of Art New York

He did, however, do much to identify and treat the disorder and his establishment doctors were the first to secure usable information about the natural history of Syphilis and its hereditary effects amongst a profoundly sickly group of infants. But it would not be the first or the last time that Syphilis and its management would be politicized and run according to an underlying agenda. Many conceded that even though it was essentially an untreatable disease, that it might be transformed into a chronically manageable ailment (perhaps a little like some less rampant cancers are today). In France, whilst prostitutes with Syphilis were being rounded up into her hospitals and her prison infirmaries, the doctors were keen to produce some evidence for the inspectors that the disease was at least nominally under some control. Quétel reports that the sicker cases were kept hidden from travelling inspectors and substituted with healthy prostitutes. So too would mouth ulcers be covered by feeding patients chocolate and vaginal chancres would be doused with bull's blood on the pretence of menstruation.[52]

Like France, Norway would adopt mandatory prostitute examinations but England's foray into a French-style punitive legislation against prostitutes would prove disastrous, provoking an angry Womens' movement headed by the militant Josephine Butler (1828–1906) whose ire was such that following the enactment of the *Contagious Diseases Act* of 1864[53] she established a group which she called the Abolitionists. The Bill had imposed a power for the Constabulary to detain and arrest any woman who they had deemed responsible for spreading the disease. If she was discovered to be infected she would then be transferred to a Lock Hospital for a minimum of 3 months without right to appeal. When the legislation was extended to the northern regions in 1866, separate groups of women in solidarity founded the *Ladies National Association for the Repeal of the Contagious Diseases Acts* to oppose the equally impossibly named *Association for Promoting the Extension of the Contagious Diseases Acts*. The two groups physically fought it out until the 1864 Act was repealed in 1886.[54]

Those sanitized hospital dispensaries were, however, also points of artistic inspirational fodder for the representation of the venereal diseases. They would prove as popular haunts for the diminutive impressionist Henri de Toulouse-Lautrec (1864–1901) as were the cabarets of the Folies-Bergère and the Moulin Rouge that he also frequented. It suited his love of prostitutes well that the riskier women were now even subjected to mandatory pelvic examinations *in locus* by inspectors visiting the local brothels and his dalliances formed the backdrop to his Bohemian lifestyle. Whilst the ladies of the night awaited their turn with the cold speculum in

---

[52] Quétel. *Ibid.* p. 223.

[53] According to Butler "*It is men, only men, from the first to the last that we have to do with! To please a man I did wrong at first, then I was flung about from man to man. Men police lay hands on us. By men we are examined, handled, doctored. In the hospital it is a man again who makes prayer and reads the Bible for us. We are had up before magistrates who are men, and we never get out of the hands of men till we die!*" She was further quoted "*God and one woman make a majority*".

[54] The *Ladies National Association for the Repeal of the Contagious Diseases Acts* developed because the original *National Association for the Repeal of the Contagious Diseases Acts* in a vote of self-defeat actually excluded women from its meetings!

the Rue des Moulin, Toulouse-Lautrec recorded their movements and sketched them as they paraded before the doctors in various stages of undress. Whilst there, he could kill two birds with one stone and the doctors could treat the Syphilis he had contracted from his most beloved of sitting models, the gentle Rosa la Rouge.[55]

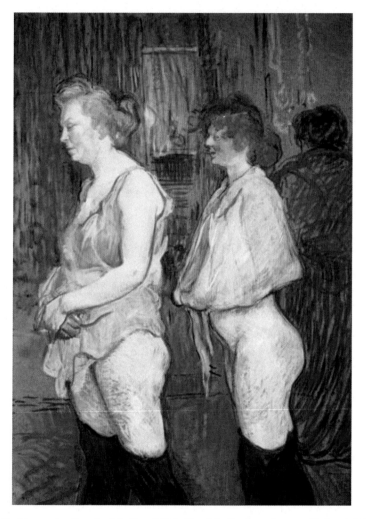

The medical inspection Rue des Moulins (1894). Henri de Toulouse-Lautrec. National Gallery of Art Washington D.C.

---

[55] Rosa la Rouge was a young red-haired girl Carmen Gaudin whom Toulouse-Lautrec first met in Montmartre in 1884. His oft used technique of painting her with her head turned away or full face still showing a shy vulnerability are both methods which display a remarkable modernity in their execution. Although she was his model, some have speculated that she was also the source of his Syphilis.

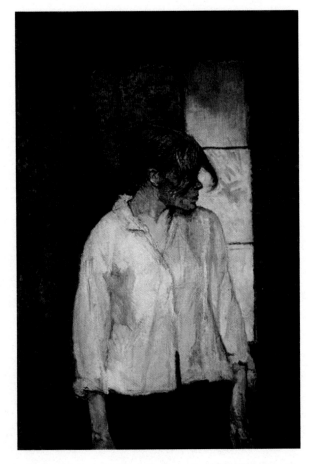

Toulouse-Lautrec H. At Montrouge (Rosa la Rouge). 1886–1887. The Barnes Foundation Phildelphia

But the less romantic notions of struggling prostitutes eking out a relatively honest living were in stark reality to the wards of the Hôpital Vaugirard brimful with the hopeless emaciated cases drawn by the Belgian satirical artist Félicien Rops (1833–1898). He had already illustrated the frontispiece of Baudelaire's dystopic *Les Fleurs du Mal* but even his personal style of erotic impressions of *fin-de-siècle* lifestyle could not sanitize the reality of a terminal syphilitic death in the isolated coldness of a Parisian infirmary. The image for the front page of Dujardin's 1909 *History of Syphilis* (a copy of his *Mors Syphilitica* now in Rops' own museum in Namur, Belgium) shows the skeletal danger that one moment's congress represents with the semblance of a disrobing woman. If that image were not enough, he crowns her with a mortifying scythe-like shaft of light that can only reflect one outcome from their union.

Syphilis had stumbled into the 20th Century, a time that would spawn an understanding of its cause and an ultimate cure. Before then, the doctors could largely do no more than just annotate the modes and their legacies of its spread and the exotic nature of its presentations awakened from prolonged periods of dormancy. In this, it would seem essentially like any medieval complaint, cloaked in secrecy, invariably lethal, aggressively destructive and lionized in poetry. But somewhere and sometime, it tempered its demeanour, becoming a more astute parasite that settled into an accepted mutual tolerance between beast and host. It was no longer a death sentence and with the advent of Penicillin it lost its spectre in a way that HIV-AIDS has just about achieved now. It has, (given the rise in worldwide deaths from congenital Syphilis), mistakenly transformed into something that provides the impression more than anything else of a public nuisance. In so doing, its literary and artistic images have also changed into something more pedestrian.

The most romantic of its reputations could only grow in the shadow of ignorance both of its cause and of its treatment even if it could never quite capture the almost pious demise of the most notable representatives of its greatest social competitors, Tuberculosis and alcoholism. The few remote cases purporting that an inflammatory response to its presence in the brain had provoked their genius were not enough to sustain its creative imagery and beyond the poster campaigns of its prevention, its link to the art world disappeared. Before it was done, however, even in the face of antibiotics with which it could be treated, registers with which it could be monitored and prophylactic methods where it could be avoided, it would contrive some men of honour stirred by their place in history as arbiters of its cause and management to conduct heinous human experimentation in its name. Perhaps the most notorious of these was the Tuskegee Experiment.

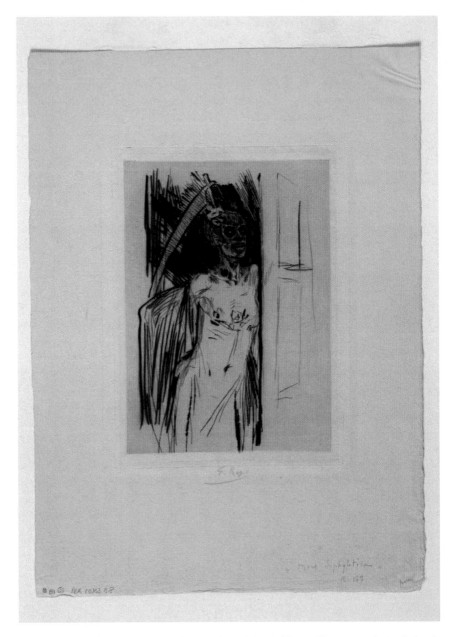

Félicien Rops, *Mors syphilitica*, 1865, drypoint, 22,2 × 16,2 cm. Courtesy and permission by Musée Félicien Rops, Province de Namur, Belgium. inv. PER E0353.1.P (© Musée Félicien Rops —Atelier de l'Imagier)

Chapter 6
Syphilitic Politics: Ethical Breaches, the Tuskegee Experiment and Beyond

> If the patient has had syphilis for 25 years without clinical disease he is to be congratulated and not treated.[*]

Abstract In the pre-microbial era, 19th Century syphilologists were busily experimenting on their patients (and even on the uninfected public) scratching them with scrapings of syphilitic and gonorrhoeal ulcers in order to see the impact of infection and cross-infection. The scientific world craved without success a reproducible animal model of Syphilis that could show longitudinally all of the stages the disease normally exhibited in humans. Into the 20th Century Tuskegee Alabama became the institute that was a byword for experimental infamy when the Public Health Service (the forerunner of the Center for Diseases Control) chose Macon Co. and its surrounds to witness over 4 decades the ravages of untreated (or deliberately poorly treated) Syphilis in an indigent Black community of men. The unethical nature of this trial only came to light after a casual conversation at a party between an academic co-worker and a journalist. From this reckoning which shed light upon this and other despicable experimentation on an uninformed cohort of vulnerable patients, spawned a National Bioethics Centre that has become an important hub of medical and ethical research. Ripples of the 'Tuskegee experiment' still permeate the psyche of the American South, contributing to a vaccine hesitancy during the COVID pandemic that disproportionately affects African Americans.

It is perhaps because Syphilis is a disease of the indigent, (sometimes spread by prostitutes and carnally conceived), that for some who made it their life's dedication, there was frequently an overwhelming urge to play fast and loose in the management of its victims both with the truth and with ethical conventions. Like cancer in a past era, the diagnosis, treatment and day-to-day impact of Syphilis would be shrouded in a double secrecy; one projected as a fear of discovery onto the outside world and the other rationalized and internalized inward to the affected case.

---

[*]Quoted as a common medical saying in Susan M. Reverby. *Tuskegee Truths: Rethinking the Tuskegee Syphilis Study*. University of North Carolina Press 2000; p. 200.

A. P. Zbar, *Syphilis*, https://doi.org/10.1007/978-3-031-08968-8_6

At the start of his reign, the Sun King Louis XIV (1638–1715) had acceded to the demands of the wife of one of his most prominent magistrates, Marie de Maupeou (1590–1681)[1] whom he had appointed Supervisor of the Lady of Charity of the Central Hospital the Hôtel Dieu and of the Hospital of the Sisters of Providence. Although an advocate for the poor, impressing upon the priesthood the necessity of the Church to become active in their care, she was sufficiently puritanical to believe that some diseases like Syphilis were retributions from God whose sufferers should expect to be denied medical aid.[2] For de Maupeou the hospitals could only be used by innocent victims of disease and were not for those acquiring their afflictions primarily through sin. *"Far from giving them help"* she wrote, *"we should add to their sufferings.*[3]*"*

The denial of treatment based upon some overarching assumptions concerning either the personality or the attributes of one entire group of those suffering from a disease would not rear its head again until the Southern physicians of Alabama would deny more than 400 African American men in Tuskegee with known latent Syphilis any treatment at all. But that story comes a little later.

The vast majority of ethical breaches in the management of patients with Syphilis would err on the side of experimental treatments often not informing prostitutes, the poverty stricken, those disadvantaged by mental illness or the incarcerated about their mendicants and inoculations. In other guise, an over eager enthusiasm would skirt ethical boundaries and transcend towards self-experimentation. Prior to any understanding of the bacterial nature of infection and still hell bent on finding out the contagious cause of disease, some would randomly infect unsuspecting medical students (or themselves) in the desperate hope to separate Syphilis from gonorrhoea and once and for all define whether they were different illnesses or the same disease. The process became something of a matter of pride for some in taunting illnesses whose origins were unknown and in the face of an inevitability of their inexorable progression once successfully inoculated. But more than pride, such self-experimentation became a symbol of scientific martyrdom and an ethical standard as yet undefined whose daring would

---

[1] de Maupeo (Mme. de Fouquet) was the wife of Francis de Fouquet.

[2] Until 1690, cases of suspected venereal disease were denied entrance to the Hôtel Dieu in Paris. Quétel quotes Regulation 1656 which created the general hospital of Paris (art. VI). *"Poverty stricken mendicants affected with leprosy or with a contagious disease or with venereal disease will not be received by the* [above named General Hospital] *and those Houses which constitute it"* [See pp. 100, 290]. This was eventually rescinded as both the Bicêtre Hospital (for men) and Saltpetrière Hospital (for women) became overloaded with cases.

[3] Marie de Maupeou. *Receuil des remèdes faciles et domèstiques ...recueilles par les orders caritabless d'une illustre et pieuse dame* 1678. [See Quétel pp. 74, 287]. When this edict was published Maupeou's name was deliberately omitted. She believed that those pious women with debauched husbands or those babies who had acquired Syphilis through an infected wet nurse should be able to be treated by local barber surgeons at the public expense. [See also *Le Théâtre des Antiquitez de Paris* (the Tracts of the Founding Churches and Chapels of the City, University and Diocese of Paris, such as the institution of Parliament, Founding University, Colleges and other Remarkable Institutions, 4 Vols) 1639 by RPF Jacques Du Bruel].

even catch the eye of the Nobel Committees.[4] For the University of Wisconsin's Professor of History and Bioethics Susan Lederer, *"The idea of self-experimentation was that it undermined accusations of research exploitation and demonstrated the nobility of the investigator".*[5]

In this sort of endeavor, the Edinburgh surgeon Benjamin Bell (1749–1806) had proudly proclaimed in his 1797 work *A Treatise on Gonorrhoea and Lues Venerea* that he had joyously observed his medical students introducing the tips of stylets (which had been soaked in syphilitic pus derived from the chancres of infected patients) hard up into their own urethras only to acquire a delayed onset of Syphilis without the transfer of gonorrhoea. He had clearly separated the diseases and although it had always been suggested that the medical students had all volunteered, Bell in his writings at least could not have seemed simultaneously either more detached or more pleased. Reading Bell's work, Jean-Francois Hernandez (1769–1835) felt compelled to inoculate the gonorrheal pus under the skin of a group of convicts in Toulon and he felt the fact that none developed Syphilis justified the intrusion. Francis Xavier Swediaur (1728–1824) was so stimulated by Bell's work that he moved from his native Austria to London and produced a rival book on venereology his magnificently entitled *Practical Observations on the More Obstinate and Inveterate Venereal Complaints* published in 1784.[6] Swediaur used it as a rallying call against the most prominent English surgeon of the day, John Hunter (1728–1793). Hunter had only recently produced his own work on venereology *A Treatise on the Venereal Disease* in 1786 after repeatedly scratching himself under the skin with a lancet soaked in the pus from a gonorrheal patient, only to have inadvertently inoculated himself with Syphilis. Swediaur remained confused, seeing one case where prostitutes afflicted with Syphilis could *"give one man the clap, another chancres and a third both at once"*. But his motivations may have been more directed at his mentor Hunter, someone who aroused the most vitriolic of jealousies and whom Swediaur regarded as *"a vain man, ignorant of the*

---

[4] Medical advance is littered with examples of self-experimenters some of whom obtained the Nobel Prize for their efforts. Such self-experimenters included Jesse Lazear who in 1900 succumbed to yellow fever after deliberately allowing himself to be bitten by an infected mosquito, Max von Pettenkoffer who in 1892 deliberately drank a soup infected with cholera bacteria and more recently Barry Marshall in 1984 who drank a concentrate of Helicobacter bacteria to induce gastritis. Constantin Levaditi injected himself with spirochaetes derived from rabbits' testicles so as to induce Syphilis but he could never successfully transfer the disease. Part V of the 1947 Nuremberg Code which emanated from the trial of Nazi experimental doctors actually requires the experimenters to participate as subjects in a study where an experimental treatment is considered dangerous. Marshall won the Nobel Prize (2005) as did Werner Forssman who performed self-cardiac catheterization studying his own heart, (1956) and Ralph Steinman who injected himself with genetically modified dendritic cells to treat his own pancreatic cancer (2011). Steinman was the only person ever awarded the Nobel Prize posthumously.

[5] Susan Lederer. *Subjected to Science. Human Experimentation in America Before the Second World War.* Johns Hopkins University Press. 1995. p. 127.

[6] Later revised into his 1798 *Traité Complet sur les Symptomes, Les Effets, la Nature et le Traitement des Maladies Syphilitiques.*

different writings and discoveries made by his contemporaries" [and who] "*can attribute to himself what should have been attributed to others*".[7]

In amongst all of this jealousy of discovery to define the natural history and mechanism of transfer of Syphilis, the French venereologist Jean Alfred Fournier would be quite definitive. "*We should not use the lancet on the healthy subject*" he wrote "*If a doctor wishes to study and to verify a scientific fact he must choose himself as the experimental subject, not the patient who entrusts himself to his care*".[8] Fournier's teacher Philippe Ricord (1800–1889) and probably France's most revered venereologist would also succumb to the temptation of treating his syphilitic patients unethically, convinced of his ability to inoculate large swathes of the population against the syphilitic 'virus' under the banner of the program dubbed '*Syphilization*' by its inventor Joseph Auzias-Turenne (1812–1870). As the novelist Charles Baudelaire had railed against the republican spirit and lyrically mused on the democratization that Syphilis once caught had engendered,[9] Ricord had actually taken him seriously.

Ricord had been persuaded to return from his home town of Baltimore after his parents had settled there to escape the French Revolution. Upon returning to Paris, he set about developing one of the largest private practices in the City largely catering to the syphilitic aristocracy. His charisma and the powerful delivery of his lectures became legendary and he acquired the reputation of a dandy with an overinflated ego. His was a life of entitlement and honour, the personal physician to Napoleon III who according to the chronicler Jules de Goncourt (himself a sufferer of Syphilis) was awarded almost one medal per Pox victim so that the "*row of ribbons on Ricord's chest was not reassuring for the state of the crowned phalluses*".[10]

As the greatest Syphilologist alive it is paradoxically possible that Ricord did more than almost anyone else to spread the disease, convinced that it was entirely non-infectious in nature during its secondary stage. Against this background, it could conversely be argued that he did possibly more than anyone else to promote its diagnosis particularly amongst the prostitutes roaming Paris, by introducing the instrument of its examination and assessment, the cold speculum. He would patiently explain in detail the need to continuously re-examine women over several days in order to avoid the missing window between infection and the first mani-festation of the small chancres that could surreptitiously develop almost unseen inside their vaginas. He was particularly graphic in his insistence on examining all the orifices of those with sexual proclivity and in introducing the world to the idea that sexual intercourse could be so much more than a penis simply penetrating a

---

[7] See J David Oriel. *The Scars of Venus. A History of Venereology*. Springer Verlag 2013: pp. 32–33.

[8] Quétel *Ibid.*. p. 142.

[9] See Chap. 5, opening Baudelaire quote.

[10] Hayden *Ibid.* p. 30. Queen Victoria once visiting Paris was met at the front of the entourage by Ricord wearing so many medals that she inquired whether he was a Field Marshal and in which campaigns he had fought.

vagina.[11] The doctors became so excited and vigorous in their examination of so many women, that it induced the new visible chancre on the examining finger which soon became known as the *'physician's chancre'*.

Ricord's practice and fame was so great that he became the dominant voice of the prevention and treatment of venereal disease for all of France and he was given *carte blanche* between 1831 and 1837 to inoculate nearly 2500 prostitutes with gonococcal pus (largely without their knowledge) in his quest to separate Syphilis and gonorrhoea. The idea that he should ever seek their permission simply never occurred to him and he indifferently had no qualms in recording the outcomes of this social experiment in his revelatory 1838 book the *Traité pratique des maladies vénériennes*. But it had not always been that easy. When he had arrived as an extern in Paris working for the great but irascible surgeon Guillaume Dupuytren (1777–1835) he was fired for daring to suggest that a procedure Dupuytren had purported to have invented was already being performed several years before in the United States and could not possibly have been devised by Dupuytren. More than this, if his relationship with Dupuytren had not already become strained, he confirmed at another proximate meeting during one of Dupuytren's presentations of a case with delirium, that the patient had actually died under Dupuytren's care. Both remarks were intolerable to the great man and Ricord was immediately dismissed, although Dupuytren did not stand in his way. Ricord recovered sufficiently by moving up the road to the Hôtel Pitié-Saltpêtrière to work with one of Napoleon's most illustrious army surgeons, the father of the field amputation, Jacques Lisfranc de St. Martin (1790–1847).[12]

For all his faults, Ricord would champion the use of the condom in France in 1826 despite vociferous protestation from the Vatican. He openly proffered its widespread use against the historical objections made from one of France's most famous letter writers Marie de Rabutin-Chantal, (the Marquise de Sévigné) (1626–

---

[11] Ricord was probably one of the first physicians to introduce the use of a mirror so that women could examine themselves. Although secondary Syphilis with its widespread popular rash and aching joint and muscle pains (as described and first categorized by Ricord) was deemed by him to be non-contagious, it is actually the most infectious stage of the illness. The idea that other forms of non-vaginal sex were possible was a particular insight of the Parisian public health expert Alexandre Jean-Baptiste Parent-Duchateley (1790–1835). Both oral and anal sex was first iterated in Parent-Duchateley's book *De la prostitution dans la ville de Paris, considérée sous le rapport de l'hygiène publique, de la morale et de l'administration* (On prostitution in the city of Paris, considered with respect to public health, morality and administration) published posthumously. Ricord in his visits to England took particular delight in the English reticence to examine the anus for signs of Syphilis and frequently found ulcerative chancres there on examinations which had been labeled previously as negative. He specifically referred to them in his notes as the *"rear entrance to this perfidious Albion"*. [Ricord P. *Lettres sur la syphilis*. Paris L'Union Médicale 1865; p. 175 and also See JD Oriel Eminent venereologists. 3. Philippe Ricord. *Genitourinary Medicine* 1989; 65: 388–93]. Under Ricord's direction, Parisian prostitutes acceded to repeated mandatory vaginal examinations by the State in their brothels (referred to as *Maisons de tolérance*) coming to refer to the speculum as the *'Government's penis'*.

[12] Ricord is reputed to have uttered during the meeting *"Amicus Plato sed magis amica veritas"* (A friend of Plato but a greater friend of truth) and reports suggest that Dupuytren became furious.

1696) who had dismissed its use. In one of her missives to her daughter the Countess of Grignon, Rabutin-Chantal describes the condom as mere *"armor against enjoyment and a spider web against danger"*.[13] It may seem today that Ricord's concepts developed in the heat of venereal Paris are archaic and that his academic output which did not produce any definitive new research, is not particularly illuminating. As much of the opportunity to diagnose Syphilis was clinical with late presentations, Ricord at least in this aspect proved himself a master.

But much of syphilitic management was also conceptual prior to any discovery of the bacillus where most held the view that not only was it a small virus but that in an age where smallpox could be controlled by vaccination that anti-Syphilis vaccination too should be possible. In France, the procedure of scratching people with small amounts of débris derived from chancres and buboes in the hope of producing a delayed pustular reaction was frequently used as a diagnostic tool in active syphilitic infection and had been used to distinguish a whole range of penile infections and ulcers.[14] Ricord's Parisian nemesis, Auzias-Turenne went one step further imploring the French Academy of Sciences to begin a program of widespread deliberate inoculation of the country's prostitutes. Without any real understanding of the complex humoral antibody and cellular responses to repeated skin injections, (either of self-derived material or material from another person), Turenne's *Syphilization* as it was so labelled was proposed for national use in those already diagnosed with Syphilis. It was designed to stimulate their immunity and in order to prevent early cases from becoming more advanced.

Although its most vociferous proponents like Auzias-Turenne referred to *Syphilization* as vaccination it was nothing more than an auto-inoculation. Somewhere along the way, however, *Syphilization* got out of hand and

---

[13] There is debate concerning the authenticity of this letter. [See Kruck Wm E. Looking for Dr Condom. Publication No.66 of the American Dialect Society USA: University of Alabama Press, 1981]. Ricord's advocacy of the use of condoms was arguably the single most effective thing he had achieved in his lifetime in the battle against venereal disease. His other great achievement was chronicling the stages of Syphilis although it is likely that he borrowed this idea in part from the work of Thierry de Héry (1505–1559) and also from Hunter's writings. In this matter, the prior divisions of Syphilis had been confusing and did not reflect the natural history of the disease where previously it had been separated into a so-called 'primitive' (or localized) disease and a constitutional (or systemic) illness. By the time Ricord retired, his own hospital the Hôpital du Midi (where he had initially intended to only spend a short time but where he worked for over 30 years), had been renamed the Hôpital Ricord but by 1903, it had been absorbed into the Hôpital Cochin. Ricord at the time became so famous that he was regularly caricatured in French magazines almost as often as Otto von Bismarck and Richard Wagner. [See Pashkov KA, *Betekhtin MS, Yevdomikov AI. Philippe Ricord—prominent venereologist of the XIXth Century. History of Medical Disciplines. 2014: 4: 13–17.*

[14] Such auto-inoculation had also been used to differentiate other sexually transmitted infections as a prior attack with syphilitic chancre was believed to render the patient immune from a secondary bout of Syphilis but not from a repeat bout either of gonorrhoea or the so-called soft chancre (later called Chancroid). It is believed that many of Ricord's patients whom he treated for Syphilis actually had Chancroid (as openly suggested in 1902 after Ricord's death by one of his students Léon Bassereau).

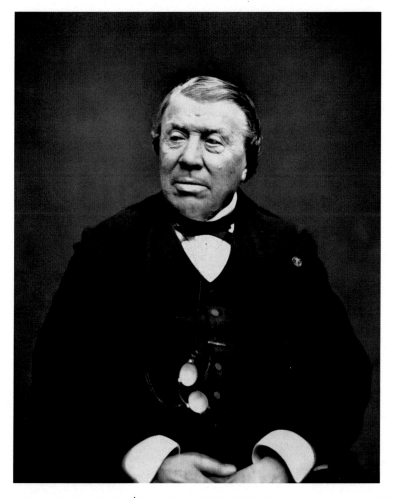

Philippe Ricord photographed by Étienne Carjat. (1828–1906) taken sometime between 1860 and 1876. Wikipedia https://en.wikipedia.org/wiki/Philippe_Ricord

Auzias-Turenne began advocating it for healthy uninfected men and women as a Syphilis prevention across the country. In 1859, he went too far, along with a dermatology colleague Camille Melchior Gilbert (1797–1866) and began deliberately infecting people with syphilitic pus insisting that the nation would benefit from his researches.[15] Although Ricord had in the beginning supported the idea, he was appalled at the concept that healthy people would be exposed to an illness for which at the time there was no cure and whose outcome was so unpredictable.

---

[15] Auzias-Turenne suggested that all prostitutes could carry a certificate of Syphilization as a measure of their health.

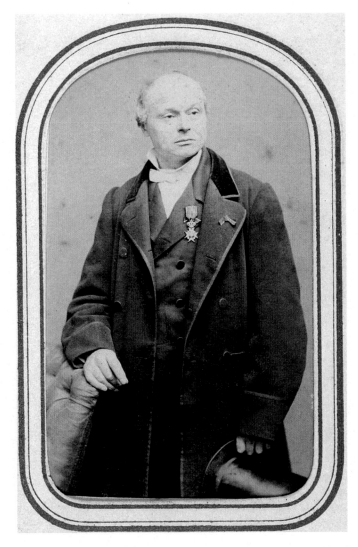

Joseph-Alexandre Auzias-Turenne 1812–1870. Wikipedia (France) https://fr.wikipedia.org/wiki/Joseph-Alexandre_Auzias-Turenne

Afterwards, Ricord went to war with Auzias-Turenne finally laying *Syphilization* (at least for France) to rest at an Academy meeting in 1852 proclaiming it to be a complete social and clinical failure.[16]

The fighting between Ricord and Auzias-Turenne took place, however, on many levels with Ricord convinced that Syphilis was a distinctly human disease and Auzias-Turenne spending his time trying to infect monkeys and rabbits. One can only imagine what these meetings were like with Auzias-Turenne displaying his monkeys with ulcers in an effort to convince the audience that they looked like the Syphilis that could be found on any infected human. Ricord taunted Auzias-Turenne and told him to "*Have the courage of one's own convictions ... [and] inoculate himself with pus from one of his monkeys' ulcers and wait for the appearance of symptoms*". Auzias-Turenne took the criticism to heart, recording it in his personal diaries but only declaring that he had done so when they were released posthumously and only then proudly attesting that he was "*the oldest syphilised person in the world*".[17] Meetings such as these settled on discrete battle lines and in Auzias-Turenne's corner was one young German doctor Ritter von Welz.

von Welz would rally to Auzias-Turenne's defence inoculating himself with the pus from a 5-day old chancre he had found on one of Turenne's monkeys and showing the small inflammatory mass that had soon developed to Ricord. von Welz could only express a delight in the fact that he might have successfully inoculated himself with Syphilis. But all ended in tragedy when in 1851 a young German Dr. Lindeman repeatedly infected himself with ulcer material until he acquired early Syphilis giving Auzias-Turenne the opportunity of treating him with his *Syphilization* program. Although the details are not known, when Lindeman died (perhaps from some allergic reaction) the scandal provoked by *Syphilization* marked its end as a social experiment.

Finally, on the 28th July 1903 the infected clitoris of a young chimpanzee was proudly displayed to an enraptured Parisian Academy as the definitive animal model of transferrable Syphilis and Ricord had been proven wrong years after both antagonists (he and Auzias-Turenne) were already dead. The little monkey was brought back for review one month later clearly showing the signs of secondary Syphilis[18] and it stimulated Albert Neisser to inoculate over 1000 monkeys and produce the disease in a new laboratory he had established in Java, Indonesia. Neisser's enthusiasm did not keep him, however, above the fray of ethical

---

[16] The Academy of Medicine officially banned *Syphilization* on 3rd August 1852. Although banned in France, *Syphilization* was utilized in Turin by Dr Sperino, Dr Gamberini in Bologna, Dr Sigmund in Vienna and in Oslo by Dr C. Boeck, [See Begin L-J. *Rapport sur un fait relatif à la syphilisation*. Bulletin de l'Académie National de Médecin. 1852; 17: 879–80 also *Sexual Cultures in Europe: Themes in sexuality*. Edited by Franz X. Eder, Lesley A. Hall and Gert Hekma. Manchester University Press, Manchester & New York 1999; p. 46].

[17] Auzias-Turenne J-A. *La syphilization*. Paris. Études Poulain d/Andecy. 1878. [See also Quétel. *Ibid* p. 113].

[18] Tertiary Syphilis does not develop in animals.

controversy, as he had already weathered a public examination of his activities after inoculating young female prostitutes with the serum of syphilitic women in 1895. An inquiry had forced him to concede that he had only succeeded in giving them active disease.[19]

Ricord straddled a period in time when the only way to diagnose Syphilis was by clinical pattern recognition. In the midst of this clinical mess he had separated Syphilis from gonorrhoea (although he did not understand the separate nature of soft Chancroid) and had ordered the illness into its defining stages. In so doing he laid the way for his students like Fournier, Charles-Paul Diday (1812–1894) and Léon Bassereau (1810–1888) to forge syphilology as a specialty in its own right with its inherent portfolio of respectable research. If he had lived long enough Ricord would have seen a disease with no clear aetiology discover the culprit microorganism. In his time there were no diagnostic tools but soon enough the diagnosis of Syphilis would yield to a simple blood test of the serum. And he would have seen the introduction of Salvarsan and a move away from mercurial rubs. He was a venereal giant at a time when intuition and experience were the principal arbiters of a successful practice. But in the end as so often happens to so many pioneering physicians, history would leave him behind.

Ricord's 'progeny' (his *fils-scièntifique*) and the natural successor of his work at the Hôtel du Midi, Jean Fournier, was (if it is possible) even more clamorous in his call to arms by France against Syphilis. Puffed up with his own importance, Fournier extolled the duty of the physicians to impose treatments and considered it fair game for the police to probe and follow sexual contacts. But even though Paris was leading the world in the annotations of all of the venereal diseases, the ethical background of much of her experimentation which had proved so suspect led almost inevitably to the next clinical question. Even if it was accepted that all patients should be treated (with such treatments as were available), what was missing from the understanding of Syphilis was the outcome of the untreated case.

---

[19] Disciplinary hearings were held concerning this 'experiment' in March 1900 charging Neisser with the performance of an activity without consent on 4 prostitutes aged between 17 and 20 years. Neisser was astonished that he should even have been questioned and was sure that the prostitutes had all acquired Syphilis by other means. After being found guilty of misconduct he was fined 300 Marks without any imposition on his license or hospital practice. Neisser who was highly regarded had already suffered restrictions in his professional ambitions most likely a result of local anti-Semitism. His demonstration as a young resident in 1879 that gonorrhoea was due to a microbe had been novel and inspiring at a time when only anthrax, relapsing fever and leprosy had been shown to have a bacterial cause. Ten months after reading about Neisser's discovery of the gonococcus, a young Romanian resident Arpad Bokai (1856–1919) injected gonorrheal pus into the urethras of 3 healthy volunteers successfully transferring acute gonorrhoea. In another dubious clinical experiment, one of Ricord's junior colleagues August Vidal de Cassis (1803–1856) took the material from a pustular breast abscess and inoculated it into a pharmacy student producing a small chancre proving that secondary Syphilis was highly infectious and forcing Ricord to publicly acknowledge his mistake. [See Perrett DB. Ethics and error: the dispute between Ricord and Auzias-Turenne over syphilisation 1847–1870. Thesis Stanford University 1977 and also Stilliams AW. Syphilisation: an episode in the evolution of venereology. Arch Dermatology Syphilology (Chicago) 1938; 37: pp. 272–8].

Could patients recover by themselves or was it inevitable that Syphilis would advance into most of the viscera and kill its host? Could expectant treatment (the *méthode expectante*) of simply watching and waiting offer a better outcome than the toxicity of the currently available therapies?

The perverse idea that not treating anyone would be justified became an obsession of an Oslo dermatologist Caesar Peter Moller Boeck (1845–1917) and withholding treatment between 1890 and 1910 at the University Hospital in 2,181 patients with early Syphilis (along the lines of the theory of expectant treatment that natural immunity would prevail over the toxicity of any therapy), he and his assistant Bruusgaard showed on tracking 473 of the patients that untreated Syphilis was indeed over time, a fatal disease.[20] So many of the patients could not be found and the Oslo study troubled some even more when Boeck and Bruusgaard had vehemently stated that they had searched for all the remaining survivors so that they could offer them the newly available and effective arsenic therapies. As Syphilis rose to epidemic proportions in Europe immediately following the First World War, France would have to amalgamate its venereal diseases watchdogs into a single cohesive entity and it had provoked the newly formed League of Nations to institute an American Cooperative Clinical Group just to deal with the problem.[21]

In the rush to understand more about disease treatment, the idea had percolated that all that was missing from the available knowledge was some uniform prospective study monitoring the progression of untreated disease over the life of the patient. To this humble end, a study was commenced by the American PHS to

---

[20] In the Boeck-Bruusgaard analysis (reported as 2 papers) the rate of neurological disease was 4 times higher than expected in the untreated Syphilis cases when compared with the non-syphilitic population and the incidence of chronic bone disease was 26 times higher comparatively in the untreated group. The findings of the study were formally presented by Trygve Gjestland in 1955 in the book *The Oslo Study of Untreated Syphilis: An epidemiologic investigation of the natural course of the syphilitic infection based upon a re-study of the Boeck-Brussgaard material*. Akademisk Forlag. The study also showed that progression of untreated Syphilis was not certain with only 25% of cases progressing to a secondary stage, 15% manifesting as cutaneous and bony tertiary disease, 14% with cardiovascular lesions and 10% with neurological degeneration.

[21] By 1918, it was estimated that there were about 800,000 new cases of Syphilis in France. It was so prevalent that it was often stated that "*A German bullet is cleaner than a whore.*" [Quoted from Colonel Care Poster Series. 1918 In American Social Hygiene Association Papers, folder 113: 6. University of Minnesota, Minneapolis-St.Paul]. The French government strove to amalgamate the Anti-Venereal Leagues of Alsace and Lorraine, the League for the Abolition of Syphilis and the French National League against Venereal Peril with Fournier's Society for the Sanitary and Moral Prophylaxis. [See Quétel. *Ibid.* p. 178]. The Health Services Division of the League of Nations (once formed) established the US Cooperative Clinical Group which functioned between 1928 and 1942 recruiting patients from Johns Hopkins University, Western Reserve University, the Mayo Clinic, the University of Pennsylvania and the University of Michigan. The group was coordinated by Pennsylvania's Professor of Dermatology John H. Stokes, Michigan's Dermatology Professor Udo Wilde, Stokes' former mentor at Johns Hopkins Joseph Earle Moore, the Mayo Clinic's Head of Dermatology Paul O'Leary, the Western Reserve's dermatologist Harold Cole and the Surgeon General Thomas Parran Jr. [See Harry M. Marks. The progress of experiment: Science and therapeutic reform in the United States 1900–1990. Cambridge Studies in the History of Medicine. 2001].

be conducted over a 6 month period to examine Syphilis and its behavior in a Black community in Alabama.[22] What followed was a subterfuge that went on for the next 40 years and which became the longest non-therapeutic study in human history. The full horrors of the *Tuskegee Study of Untreated Syphilis in the Negro Male* (as it became openly dubbed by its researchers) would only become apparent when a whistleblower disgusted by the lack of ethical standard employed by its researchers informed the National Press in 1972. The fallout repercussions would change the nature of human experimentation and its conduct in the United States and around the world.

Although the story of Tuskegee has been frequently told and from many different perspectives and with differing agendas (as any retrospective assessment of history can be told), it bears some repeating. No such assessment can of course examine it divorced from its moral and ethical perspectives and even though some respected African American physicians had argued dispassionately for its scientific worth[23] it would be unlikely in today's day and age of data scrutiny to pass muster as a valid piece of scientific work. It even lacked any informed consent from its participants which would fall at the publication acceptance level anyway. Our understanding of these events and their surrounds are particularly influenced by the seminal work of Columbia's Allan M. Brandt in his influential article *Racism and Research*[24] or James H. Jones' book *Bad Blood*[25] and Wellesley College's Susan M. Reverby most notably in her *Examining Tuskegee.*[26]

Macon county Alabama was deemed the best area to be the seat of a study begun in 1932 and conducted by the United States Public Health Service (PHS) under the auspices of the Surgeon General to ask the question what was the 'natural history' of untreated latent (and presumably non-contagious) Syphilis in the Black male. Now there are so many assumptions just in this opening statement which we shall

---

[22] Like many of these studies preceding work had been conducted between 1929 and 1931 by the Julius Rosenwald Foundation initially examining the incidence of seropositivity (a positive Wasserman blood test) amongst Blacks in the southern United States. The Fund had budgeted $50,000 for the study singling out the communities of Macon Co. Alabama; Scott Co. Mississippi; Tipton Co. Tennessee; Glynn Co. Georgia; Pitt Co. North Carolina and Albemarle Co. Virginia. Financial devastation of the Rosenwald Fund by the Depression had forced it to curtail its philanthropic contributions primarily examining the health of the African American population.

[23] [See Charles J. McDonald. *The contribution of the Tuskegee Study to medical knowledge.* Journal of the National Medical Association 1974; 66(1): pp. 1–7]. Medical publication of trial data is subject to strict regulations and this would not have been published today without institutional board ethical approval and configuration of patient informed consent which now is conferred in accordance with the CONSORT (**Cons**olidated **S**tandards of **Rep**orting **T**rials) international guidelines governing the conduct of randomized controlled trials and their reporting. A 25 point ethical checklist was introduced in 2010.

[24] Allan M. Brandt. *Racism and research: the case of the Tuskegee Syphilis Study.* The Hastings Center Report. 1978; 8(6): pp. 21–29.

[25] James H. Jones. *Bad Blood. The Tuskegee Syphilis Experiment.* Free Press 1982.

[26] Susan M Reverby. *Examining Tuskegee. The infamous syphilis study and its legacy. (The John Hope Franklin Series in African American History and Culture).* University of North Carolina Press 2009.

come to presently. The study ran as a prospective follow-up (monitoring the outcomes of patients as they went along), recruiting some 400 African American males and comparing their outcomes with 200 non-Syphilitic Black men. It examined each one clinically, drawing blood for regular Wasserman reaction serology testing and over time in those sufficiently compliant obtaining through spinal tap needle insertions into their backs, the requisite spinal fluid[27] in order to determine if there were features of neurosyphilis. All of the cases who under follow-up died during the conduct of the study were to be submitted to a post-mortem (autopsy) examination and for this privilege, in 1933 shortly after commencement of the study the funeral and burial expenses (of $50 per head) were covered by the Milbank Memorial Fund.

Patients were not told of their diagnosis or progress short of referring to their condition as one of "*bad blood*" which although a euphemism for Syphilis also encapsulated many other diagnoses prevalent in African American communities. At a time when Penicillin became available (more widely in the early 1950s) and where there had been clear evidence of its efficacy even in advanced cases of Syphilis), antibiotic therapy for some patients was actively withheld by order of the officials of the study and acting under the imprimatur of the PHS and its spinoff, Atlanta's Center for Disease Control (the CDC).[28] The 'treatments' such as they were, (including pink pills tinged with a red tincture and composed of aspirin and supplemental tonics), were coordinated in their administration by an African American nurse, Eunice Verdell Rivers Laurie (1899–1986) recruited specifically for this purpose. The study continued for 4 decades up until 1972 until one of its researchers and investigators Peter Buxtun so uncomfortable with the ethics of the trial and unable to receive adequate responses to his questions from the study hierarchy, discussed the matter with an Associated Press reporter. After this it became a powerful national news item and forced an immediate shut down of the trial.[29]

Tuskegee has become a byword for unethical research standards, resulting in Senate hearings that afterwards provoked legislative changes in American clinical

---

[27] The procedure is called a lumbar puncture and is designed to examine the cells and the Wasserman reactivity of the cerebrospinal fluid. The technique although routinely performed for suspicious meningitis is painful and has complications the commonest of which is a significant post-procedural headache. Some reports have suggested that the subjects particularly feared spinal taps as it was thought that they drew away some of their procreative powers.

[28] The US PHS was originally chartered in 1798 as the Marine Health Service with an interest in the health of navy mariners and it became a national health service with jurisdiction over clean water and sanitation establishing a Surgeon General by the end of the 19th Century. It first conducted biomedical research in 1887 openly advocating clinical research on captive populations such as prisoners and inmates of mental asylums. [See Ralph Chester Williams. *United States Public Health Service*]. In 1908, Congress established the Division of Venereal Diseases at the PHS].

[29] Jean Heller's article was filed in *The Washington Star* on 26th July 1972 as "*Syphilis Victims in US Study went untreated for 40 years*".

research through its Belmont Report [30] and that altered the nature of informed consent worldwide. It had fathered conceptual tenets of justice and had defined the capacity of research to do either harm (maleficence) or good (beneficence). In its wake, it initiated hospital and University institutional review boards and ethics committees, it established American Biomedical Ethics as a distinct discipline, it partially resolved the Tuskegee dispute in a class action out of court settlement and it spawned a Presidential apology.[31]

How on earth did this happen? I am neither an historian nor a bioethicist and one can only broadly analyze the chronology of events as reported and their general social impact. Macon County was selected because it represented a typical southern region with an 80% Black predominance where most lived in abject poverty, where the majority were illiterate and where they could be followed with the semblance of the provision of health care. It was the home of Booker T. Washington's (1856–1915) experiment that had established the Tuskegee Institute to examine the progress of 'Negro disease' and which had forged its local hospital (the John A. Andrew Memorial) staffed with its requisite Black doctors, Black nurses and Black researchers.[32] The initial work put out by the group had already produced disturbing reading. Some 36% of African Americans had tested positive with their Wasserman test and with this single finding even if it was not the stated aim of the PHS, Syphilis had potentially become a Black problem. In the aftermath of this shocking data, the Rosenwald Fund voted to withdraw its financial support and this decision may have inadvertently stimulated the Government to obstinately pursue

---

[30] The Belmont Report (30th September 1978) established the ethical guidelines for the conduct of human research in the United States and set in stone the principles of respect for individuals, beneficence and justice as the cornerstones of biomedical research practice as well as the basic nature of informed consent. Its basis cited the Nazi doctors' trial in Nuremberg (called the Subsequent Nuremberg Trials) in 1946–7 of 20 medical defendants accused of involvement in human experimentation. [See Weindling PJ. *Nazi Medicine and the Nuremberg Trials: From Medical War Crimes to Informed Consent*. Palgrave Macmillan 2005 and also Vivien Spitz. *Doctors from Hell*. Sentient Publications. 2005]. All research now must comply with the Helsinki Declaration formulated in 1975 concerning the Ethical Principles for Medical Research Involving Human Subjects.

[31] Each participant had been paid $25 with occasional $1–$2 supplements. Leroy E. Burney (1906–1998) who served as Surgeon General between 1956 and 1961 (and who in retirement served on the Board of the Milbank Memorial Fund), ensured that each subject received a signed certificate. On July 23rd 1973, Attorney Fred Gray acting for 41/112 subjects still alive and 48 heirs of those who had already died, filed a $1.8 Billion lawsuit against the United States, the State of Alabama, the Department of Health Education and Welfare (the HEW), the PHS, the CDC, the State Board of Health Alabama, the Milbank Memorial Fund and against individual physicians involved in the Tuskegee Study. An out of court settlement was made for $10 Million in December 1974 allocating each of the subjects $37,500, their heirs and families $15,000, $16,000 for controls and $5,000 for the families of control cases. Gray was so confident about winning that he remortgaged his house to pay for the initial legal costs.

[32] Booker T. Washington became the first leader of the Tuskegee Institute school, (the forerunner of Tuskegee University) raising money from private philanthropists to improve local health services in the American south and attracting the agricultural scientist George Washington Carver (1880s?—1943) to head its Agricultural Department of Research.

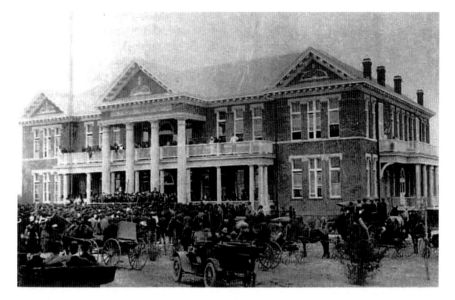

Opening of the John A. Andrew Hospital in 1913. (Reprinted with permission Tuskegee University Archives Tuskegee, AL)

its interests in the non-treatment of Syphilis in such a vulnerable group. This would have been spurred on almost certainly by the prevailing view (in the absence of any real scientific evidence) that somehow Black and White Syphilis were different diseases.[33]

---

[33] The impression was that tertiary Syphilis in African Americans was more cardiovascular in its presentation and that a neurosyphilis presentation was uncommon. The Johns Hopkins researcher Joseph Earle Moore was quoted saying that *"Syphilis in the Negro was in many respects almost a different disease from Syphilis in the White"*. [See Joseph Earle Moore. *Penicillin in Syphilis.* Springfield Ill. Charles C. Thomas 1946]. The organizing doctors were shocked to find such a high rate of serum positivity for Syphilis with Macon County's rate exceeding the other counties tested. The use of anti-Syphilis treatments (available for those with early Syphilis who were being treated outside of the Study) was also quite different across the counties. Macon County for example had over the time of the study the least number of administrations of arsenicals compared with the other counties although it had the highest number of mercury rubs administered per capita. Many had used 'anthropological' arguments of differences in racial drug responsiveness, race-related illnesses and increased disease susceptibility to suggest that the American Negro was doomed to extinction. As evidence for this view, researchers have cited the higher incidence in African Americans of sickle cell anemia, enzyme deficiencies which affect anti-malarial drug sensitivity, differences in metabolism compared with Caucasians of cardiac medications (such as ACE inhibitors used in hypertension and heart failure) and an inherent reported immunity to malarial infection with a lack of effect of malarial therapy in advanced Syphilis. [See Melbourne Tapper. *An Anthropopathology of the American Negro. Anthropology Genetics and the New Racial Science. 1940–1952.* Social History of Medicine August 1997; 10: pp. 263–81 and also Jay F. Schamberg, Carroll S. Wright. *Treatment of Syphilis.* New York Appleton 1932: p. 525; Joseph Earle Moore. *The Modern Treatment of Syphilis.* 2nd Edn. Springfield Ill. Charles C. Thomas. 1947. See also the

In amongst the protocols of the study, there might have been, however, some laudable elements. At its commencement there was scant information of the developing nature of syphilitic presentations at a time when treatments were toxic and when the infectivity of some of the different stages was not known nor the safety and efficacy of treatment in those with advanced disease who already had peripheral organ damage. But once Penicillin became widely available in the late 1940s and particularly after John Mahoney had shown its ability to cure early Syphilis in his Staten Island studies,[34] no reasonable person would have felt comfortable denying Macon County's Study subjects any sort of potentially curative treatments. Although over time, most of the men found their way to Penicillin, most also had inadequate courses of therapy and there is enough correspondence evidence with the PHS to show that doctors were frequently rebuked for going 'off the reservation' and actually treating their patients at all.

The lack of exact numbers, the difficulty with old autopsy data to determine the precise causes of death, the falsely positive nature of some of the blood tests and the fact that some in the control group subsequently acquired Syphilis, will always make it impossible to state with any degree of accuracy the number of men who might have died through lack of treatment. But there was clearly a difference in the overall mortality from Syphilis (over the non-syphilitics) and in the morbid affectations of serious cardiac and neurologic disease in those with the illness. The poor conduct of the study belied the value of continuing to collect comparatively useless data which at the expense of these men had shown what was already known; namely, that Syphilis (Black or White) was a morbid and a mortal disease.[35] The repeated decisions in the face of overwhelming evidence of the dangers of lack of treatment seemed stubborn, capricious and immoral.

Even though the whole conduct of the trial must have bothered many people there was rarely a rumbling within the PHS hierarchy through many trial managers and numerous field agents.[36] It finally took one investigator from San Francisco, Peter Buxtun to become the whistleblower divulging the information to a young AP reporter Edith Lederer at a dinner party who then sent it to the more senior reporter Jean Heller at her Washington office. The rest as they say, was history. As for Buxtun, a man who started out with investigative questionnaires for his patients and who wrote his reports back to the PHS with a demonstrative flair, it was in his very

---

evocatively entitled *The Biology of the Negro* by Julian Herman Lewis. Chicago. Chicago University Press.1942].

[34] John F. Mahoney, RC Arnold, A Harris. *Penicillin treatment of early syphilis: A preliminary report*. American Journal of Public Health. December 1943; 33: pp. 1387–91.

[35] Precedent had already been provided concerning the causes of death in Syphilis by a study performed by Paul D. Rosahn at Yale in 1940 whose findings could have obviated the need for the Tuskegee study. [See Paul D. Rosahn. *Autopsy studies in syphilis*. Washington D.C. PHS 1949 Publication].

[36] In 1965, Irwin Schatz, a Henry Ford Hospital cardiologist, had also formally expressed concerns to the CDC without receiving a reply and a statistician Bill Jenkins had even written a concerning editorial on the matter to the New York Times and the Washington Post. After their publication, however, nothing happened.

nature. He was a member of the National Rifle Association, born in Prague and speaking a fluent German, perhaps pre-requisites that proved integral to his response to Tuskegee. Most likely, the 1948 Code which came out of the Nuremberg trials of the Nazi doctors during World War II would have in their German transcripts seemed to him disturbingly ironic. When Buxtun had left the PHS to study law in 1968, his personal disquiet discussing Tuskegee with law professors and moralists (even before the concepts of bioethics had fully emerged), became persistent. Repeated letters over 7 years to the Venereal Division of the CDC in Atlanta had gone unanswered and one can only imagine his frustration and his need to speak to someone. By that time, 74 of the subjects remained alive and even the Department of Health, Education and Welfare, (the HEW) launching its own internal investigation had recognized that the study had been '*ethically unjustified*'.[37]

Despite almost all of the subjects ultimately receiving their Penicillin, its beneficial effects seemed uncertain and its impact only appeared to cloud the issue even more. Before its use, Tuskegee's lead researcher Raymond Vonderlehr (1897–1973) after showing the deleterious effects on the life tables of untreated men, had pleaded with his superior Taliaferro Clark, (1867–1948) the Director of the Venereal Diseases Division of the PHS, to extend the study for another 5 years, callously convinced that he could detect even more pathology. His enthusiasm would reward Vonderlehr with the Directorship after Clark's retirement and it would embed Tuskegee and all its tendrils firmly into the functioning arm of the PHS with Tuskegee's own men insinuating themselves into the Venereal Diseases leadership group for decades. This level of support could never be construed as accidental or fortuitous. And after Penicillin, in a woolly hind-sight assessment of the study whose stated aim was the denial of treatment, of all the patients under Macon County care admitted for Penicillin therapy, almost none had received a full course. The only advantage it would seem of being a study subject was that it could exempt one from Army service.[38]

As for the publications, (some 13 in all published between 1936 and 1973), they make chilling reading and it is hard as a medical academic to remain detached in these papers from their consequence. They read like normal medical articles can except that there are racial assumptions that are made that feel throughout as if there is '*something off*'. The Oslo paper had suggested that there might have been many

---

[37] Final report of the Tuskegee Syphilis Study Ad Hoc Advisory Panel. Department of Health, Education and Welfare (HEW) Washington D.C. 1973.

[38] Men in the Tuskegee Study were excluded from the 1941 draft after Pearl Harbor. Thomas Parran Jr. (1892–1968) had already been the Director of the Venereal Diseases Division of the PHS and went on to become US Surgeon General in 1936. He was also one of the principal heads of the US Cooperative Clinical Group set up to examine Syphilis management after World War 1. A diagnosis of Syphilis in African Americans did not preclude their entrance into the Armed Forces whereas it prohibited White enrolment. [See Allan M. Brandt. *No Magic Bullet*. New York Oxford University Press 1987; p. 116 also McBride David. *From TB to AIDS: Epidemics among urban Blacks since 1900*. Albany SUNY Press 1991].

cases of '*spontaneous cure*' but it had recognized within those with latent disease that Syphilis was sufficiently serious as to produce a fatal outcome when untreated. And yet is spawned rather than spurned Tuskegee. In the first Tuskegee paper in 1936, Vonderhlehr had shown the higher death rate when compared with the non-syphilitic controls and when some of the control group of men ultimately were found to have had Syphilis themselves, the effect on mortality would have been even more stark. Vonderlehr had shown the disease where everyone else had already suspected it, in the bones, the eyes and the gut and what is more he had shown that African American men were not immune to neurological involvement and degeneration.[39]

Ten years later their researcher John Heller (1905–1989) and his colleagues had confirmed that untreated Syphilis conferred a shorter life expectancy particularly if it was acquired in middle age[40] and in its title, there appear to be no qualms in observing unmanaged cases. One of the Tuskegee Institute directors, Austin Diebert dispassionately reported on the central nervous system and cardiovascular consequences of untreated disease[41] and this was calmly followed by an article from Jesse Jerome Peters (the study's longest serving medical expert) on the autopsy data.[42] Just before then, Sid Olansky, (1914–2007) one of Tuskegee's most active published researchers (and also one of its most vociferous defendants after the negligence by the study came to public light), had himself shown that the differences in the outcomes between the Syphilis cases and the non-syphilitics was not a measure of their deprivation. Both groups (he contested) had been equally disadvantaged by socioeconomics, each with similar housing, education and impoverishment.[43] The accrual of such information just proved more and more disconcerting and yet it remained unchecked. By the time Olansky was reporting the differences between the groups in 1956, his data were so jumbled that in the

---

[39] The first paper of the Study was Vondehrlehr RA et al. *Untreated Syphilis in the Male Negro.* Journal Venereal Diseases and Information 1936; 17: 260–5.

[40] Heller JR Jr, Bruyere PT. *Untreated Syphilis in the Male Negro. II. Mortality during 12 years of observation.* J Venereal Diseases and Information. 1946; 27: 34–38.

[41] Diebert AV, Bruyere MC. *Untreated Syphilis in the Male Negro. III. Evidence of cardiovascular abnormalities and other forms of morbidity.* Journal of Venereal Diseases and Information. 1946; 27: 301. The 4th paper was Pesare Pasquale J, Bauer TJ, Gleeson GA. *Untreated Syphilis in the Male Negro: Observations of abnormalities over 16 years.* American Journal of Syphilology. 1950; 34: 201–3 and the 5th paper was by Rivers Eunice, Schuman SH, Simpson L and Sid Olansky. *Twenty years of follow-up experience in a long-range medical study.* Public Health Reports 1953; 68: 391–5. The 6th report was Shafter JK, Usilton LJ, Gleeson GA. *Untreated Syphilis in the male Negro: Prospective study of the effect on life expectancy.* Public Health Reports. 1954; 69: 684–90.

[42] Peters JJ et al. *Untreated Syphilis in the Male Negro. Pathologic findings in syphilitic and non-syphilitic patients.* J Chronic Diseases 1955; 1: 127–148.

[43] Olansky S, Simpson L, Schuman SH. *Untreated Syphilis in the Male Negro. Environmental health factors in Tuskegee Study.* Public Health Reports 1954; 69: 691–8.

article title he could only compare Syphilis cases with what he had labelled '*pre-sumably non-syphilitic cases*'.[44]

How are we to interpret this shameful episode in American cultural and racial history? There are reams of articles, documentaries, plays, telemovies, musicals and even jazz interpretations that stylistically embrace its poetic narratives; each reflecting on how Tuskegee has become absorbed into the complex racial struggle that still so occupies the American psyche more than 150 years after the jingoistic impression of a defining end to its Civil War.

To examine Tuskegee, there are many paradigms and each will be approached from perhaps a distinctly partisan perspective, pushing it at each end with individual bias. History is like that sometimes, defined more by our own culturally interpretative impressions of what we imagine happened rather than by its factual chronology and with no singular reflection ever able to divorce itself from the restricting prism of the examiner. It is history's Heisenberg principle. No amount of objective rumination can perhaps ever supersede the subjectivity of a single rear-vision view. In one guise, Tuskegee will have its factualists caught up in the infrastructure of its lies and its deceptions. Here there is much fodder for those who might feel aggrieved and whose imperative is to prevent its recurrence. Those integrally involved could never really reconcile themselves to the fact that they were coercive in their patient recruitment and duplicitous in their explanations (if any) to others who were never placed in a position to provide something even remotely resembling informed consent. The conducive carrot of special burial rites bankrolled by New York's Milbank Memorial Fund for the opportunity of performing post-mortem dissections on those who had died under study may seem like the most practical of fiscal transactions. For some too poor to enter consecrated ground and who might otherwise have been relinquished to the common ossuary of the burial grounds of any city's Potter's Field, in its most basic form it more likely appears as a simple bribe. But in a broader historical context of the social and cultural fears of dismemberment after death (and for some a crude disruption of the soul), it transcended into something abhorrent.

---

[44] Olansky S et al. *Untreated Syphilis in the Male Negro. X. Twenty years of clinical studies of untreated syphilitics and presumably non-syphilitic groups.* J Chronic Disease 1956; 4: 177–85. Other papers in the series included: Schuman Stanley H. et al. *Untreated Syphilis in the male Negro: Background and current status of patients in the Tuskegee Study.* Journal of Chronic Diseases November 1955; 2: pp. 543–558 (9th paper); Olansky S et al. *Untreated Syphilis in the male Negro: 22 years of serological observation in a selected syphilis study group.* AMA Archives of Dermatology May 1956; 73: pp. 519–522 (11th paper); Donald Rockwell, AR Yobs, MB Moore Jr. *The Tuskegee Study of untreated syphilis: the 30th year of observation.* Archives of Internal Medicine December 1961; 114: pp. 792–798 (12th paper) and Joseph G. Caldwell, EV Pierce, AL Schroeter and GF Fletcher. *Aortic regurgitation in the Tuskegee Study of untreated Syphilis.* Journal of Chronic Diseases March 1973; 26: pp. 187–194 (13th and final paper).

Like any guard who served willingly on the barbed wire lines of a Nazi concentration camp (as Daniel Jonah Goldhagen might have us believe),[45] history for these people after that point will always be a fretful journey between repentance and obstinate self-justification. It would be no different for nurse Eunice Rivers (never called to testify in front of a judiciary committee), who one imagines privately struggled to reconcile everything her nursing ethics would have told her should have guided her daily life with the reality that her behaviour at almost all points contravened those stated principles. Rivers even now escapes scrutiny (although in some ways she remains the most tragic of figures), clouded by her own convivial and complicit silence. It is the abstracted rationalization of any body of work that openly displayed her pride in being rewarded by the HEW with a medal for her meritorious service or that saw her remembered fondly by her patients even when they realized that she was actively preventing their care.[46] More than this, it was her task to secure each autopsy, a benchmark that she would personally chide herself about whenever one escaped her net.

The same distorted level of despair appears in the notations of one of Tuskegee's principal researchers, Sidney Olansky when he was confronted by an open letter from a Georgia physician Count Gibson (1921–2002) back in 1955.[47] Gibson, an Associate Professor of Medicine at Virginia Medical College had questioned the ethical basis of what Olansky was doing after he had heard Olansky speak at a medical meeting. In his private letter to Olansky, Gibson cited his impressions of the codes of Hippocrates, Maimonides and the existent tenet of ethics of the American Medical Association. But none of this could move Olansky. It would never be enough for such a person whose guiding hands are the ethical principles of patient care to leave it as Olansky did in his reply letter. In it, Olansky recognized that the study was *"callous and unmindful of the welfare of the individual"* and rather meekly that it too had given him pause. Those who do not acknowledge a moral flaw can potentially be educated as to its centrality and importance. On the

---

[45] See Daniel Jonah Goldhagen. *Hitler's Willing Executioners. Ordinary Germans and the Holocaust.* Vintage Books 1997. (Hitlers willige Vollstrecker: Ganz gewöhnliche Deutsche und der Holocaust-German Edition). Goldhagen's controversial thesis was that the Holocaust could not have occurred (despite denial) without a willing participation of ordinary Germans already invested in genocide through a cultivated national heritage of established anti-Semitism. By extension this would be a necessary requirement for any allied or comparative atrocity such as Tuskegee which could only occur on a background where there was an entrenched pre-existing racial stereotyping.

[46] Rivers was awarded the Oveta Culp Hobby Medal in 1958 the highest award for HEW meritorious service. Hobby (1905–1995) was the first Secretary of the US Department of Health and the inaugural Director of the Womens' Army Corps. Although Hobby stepped down after batches of Polio vaccine had included live unattenuated virus and where several vaccinated children had died, President Eisenhower put her name forward in 1960 as the first female candidate to run for the US Presidency. Hobby declined the invitation.

[47] Letter to Sid Olansky from Count Gibson 28th May 1955. [See Reverby. *Ibid.* pp: 70–71, 282].

other side, it is perhaps a worse moral problem to recognize the immorality of what you are engaged in and then to do nothing about it.[48]

Beyond this *'Factual Tuskegee'* lies the *'Racial Tuskegee.* Such an abuse of medical experimentation cannot occur without some historical and cultural pre-conditioning. In America, the racial divide permitted almost any *"contingency of place"* (as Susan Reverby so aptly defines it)[49] for conduct of the study and for the analysis of Negro health. Macon County Alabama during the Depression repre-sented a perfect storm for experimenters with its top-heavy African American population, its prevalence of inherently poor, its high rate of illiteracy and its segregated education and health services. Tuskegee's Negroes would be seduced by the promise of health care populated by Black doctors and Black nurses purpose-fully designed just for them which traded the guise of service at least in this experiment for unheralded observation of the effects of no service at all.[50]

The Tuskegee Institute although now seared into the American consciousness by its first name, was somehow no longer a place but more an embodiment of anything essentially unethical. But Tuskegee's origin was so different, crystallized as it was in the mind of its founder Booker T. Washington one of the last Black community leaders to have been born into slavery. For Washington, Tuskegee was a visible reminder that was in opposition to the Jim Crow legislation enacted after the Post-Bellum Reconstruction period where the States had shored up and enshrined racial segregation in America into law. America's apartheid society that separated the schools, hospitals and water fountains of its cities would not be swept aside until the beginnings of the Civil Rights Movement. Washington, using the softer approach to democratize Black lives, would never live to see it.[51]

---

[48] Olansky in his reply to Gibson had astonishingly confessed that *"all the things that bothered you, bothered me"* [See Reverby *Ibid* p 71] even though later he believes that he had helped the Tuskegee subjects immeasurably. This comment is extraordinary as it attests to the fact that the more personal the study became, the more (not the less) permissible was the violation of their trust. Olansky for his part never suggested publicly that he had significant doubts concerning the ethical conduct of the study. As for Gibson, he was instrumental in setting up the concept of community health centres for poor communities particularly in Boston, the Mississippi Delta and the San Joaquin Valley in California.

[49] Reverby, Susan M. *Examining Tuskegee. Ibid* p. 13.

[50] Today, the demographics of Macon County remain essentially unchanged. In the 2010 Census, of the 21,452 residents, 82.6% are African American with a current median household income that is 40% of the national average and with nearly one-third of the population living below the poverty line.

[51] Washington's approach to work within the Jim Crow legislation was enunciated in a famous speech gently called the Atlanta Compromise delivered in 1895 (and which ultimately spawned the opposing more militant NAACP bent on establishing equal rights over the simpler concept of equality under the law). The Jim Crow laws enacted by the southern states commencing in the 1880s cemented racial segregation and would only be swept away with the personal and property Civil Rights Acts enacted under President Lyndon Johnson in 1964 and 1968. Paradoxically, it might sadly be argued that Washington's more passive approach may have provided more fertile ground for the institution of the Tuskegee Study. [See Louis Harlan. *The Secret Life of Booker T.*

Washington's vision was far removed from the response the word 'Tuskegee' invokes now and through his Institute and University he had coordinated Black schools and literacy programmes and a distinctly vibrant Black economy around the existent segregated principles. With this philosophy he had succeeded in raising a large amount of money through his connections to the oil magnate Henry Rogers, (1840–1909) the Sears and Roebuck president Julius Rosenwald (1862–1932) and Kodak's George Eastman (1854–1932). The thanks he received for this endeavour were to be tainted as a sufferer of Syphilis himself when his premature death from high blood pressure was mislabelled as "*death from racial characteristics*" (a euphemism for advanced Syphilis).[52] Within this *Racial Tuskegee* there is the pervasive social Darwinism that purported the perverse skeletal inferiority of the Black race with many convinced that Blacks were inherently doomed to an early extinction, if only because of a basic metabolic inferiority and an associated increased susceptibility to disease. These biological arguments would be viciously used to define the communitarian threat of their integration and the impression of a contaminating genetic degeneracy should mixture of the races (miscegenation of the Negro) ever be contemplated.[53] And its prevailing views would generate the most hateful articles published in esteemed medical journals. The idea was so pervasive that it had some like Baltimore's Professor of Biology Raymond Pearl (1879–1940) examining the weights of the Negro brain[54] and others adamantly proclaiming the veracity of the Black sexual appetite.[55]

Then there is the '*Medical Tuskegee*' that presents its scientific face through the power of repeat publication and which recruited its willing co-authors each of whom in silence acquiesced to its basic aims and principles. By any standards, the study shows so many flaws that no journal today even outside of its ethical constraints would likely publish. This is not to decry its ethical structure (or lack thereof) and to merely suggest that criticisms to the study would or should be almost entirely logistical. But at least it is of value to list the flaws of the studies with the principal problem of study contamination. Some amongst the control group clearly had Syphilis. Some of the syphilitic recruits included those with early

---

Washington. In Washington in Perspective, Essays of Louis R Harlan edited by Raymond W. Smock. Jackson University Press of Mississippi 1988: pp. 110–132].

[52] The rumour that Washington suffered from untreated Syphilis was finally put to rest when his medical records were examined, revealing a premature death from hypertension and kidney failure. [See AP's Alex Dominguez *Washington Post* May 5, 2006. *Booker T. Washington's Death Revisited*].

[53] Homer M. Folkes. *The Negro as a Health Problem.* Journal of the National Medical Association. October 8th 1910; 55: p. 1246.

[54] Raymond Pearl. *The weight of the Negro brain.* Brain Anthropology 1934; 80: 431–4.

[55] [See Carly Paul S. and Wenger O.C. *The prevalence of syphilis in apparently healthy Negroes in Mississippi.* Journal of the American Medical Association June 4th 1930; 94: pp. 1826–9; quoted in Reverby *Ibid.* p. 27]. The threat of being 'over-run' by the mixing of the races had led Marvin L. Graves to argue in the Southern Medical Journal (a journal to my distress I have also published in!) the case for Black emasculation. [See Marvin L. Graves. *A menace to the health of the White race.* Southern Medical Journal 1916; 9: pp. 407–11].

eminently treatable disease and some most likely had syphilitic exposure but there was no reason to presume them either latent or contagious. Others had different non-syphilitic cardiovascular and neurological diseases and happened to be Wasserman-Bordet positive. Still more had been partially treated with mercurials, Penicillin and other therapies.

On this background, most had no real confirmatory testing (short of exposure to their naïve immunological system as evident by a simple standing blood test). Furthermore, there was frequently no real pathological proof of syphilitic injury, an effect compounded by inadequate postmortem data. By all accounts each subgroup had no real fidelity (as one might so categorize it) that any non-treatment effect could be meaningfully compared. This is not to say that as a scientific experiment it was useless, but more perhaps next to useless where almost none of the anticipatory questions raised by the study in the first instance, ended up being adequately answered. Should latent disease be treated? How infectious is untreated latent disease? Who is and is not eradicated? Is advanced visceral disease ameliorated by treatment at all? Does Black and White Syphilis differ in its behaviour and treatment? At the end even if we ourselves would be detached observers, none of us would be any the wiser.

And perhaps although not finally, there is the *'Mythical'* or the *'Folkloric Tuskegee'*. It sits in memory differently to how it unfolded and many still mistakenly identify it as a direct syphilitic inoculation of an unsuspecting public. It solidly forms also in vivid memory in Tuskegee's Human and Civil Rights Multicultural Center (founded by Attorney Fred Gray), in the memorialized names of each one of its victims etched into its floor and in the video-memoirs of the subjects and their families. Each living memoir has a decidedly more astringent potency than any written affidavit; a lesson learned under the constraints of time from the witness testimonies of victims of the Holocaust. The symbolic Tuskegee is how we imagine Tuskegee. The historical Tuskegee is hopefully what we might do with that knowledge. As opposed to this there is a counter-history (or as anthropologist Richard Shweder prefers), a counter-narrative that will reflect the complexity of any medical study (and hence its interpretation) and which will lead to a more layered or nuanced response that might amongst all the unethical practice still identify some benefit.[56]

But Tuskegee would not be the final arbiter of exploitative syphilitic science. In the case of John Charles Cutler (1915–2003) at one time the Acting Director of the Venereal Diseases section of the PHS, such ethically questionable experimentation on unsuspecting patients became almost habitual. Cutler who had trained in the most ethical of environments at the Venereal Diseases Research Center on Staten Island, had graduated to work closely with Olansky on the Tuskegee study. Forged possibly with a perverse moral persuasion, Cutler had coordinated a 1954 study on inmates at the Sing Sing penitentiary in upstate New York in which he inoculated

---

[56] [See Richard Shweder. *The idea of moral progress. Bush vs Posner vs Berlin.* Philosophy of Education Year Book. Urbana Ill. Philosophy of Education Society. 2003; pp. 29–56].

them with attenuated material derived from the testicles of syphilitic rabbits. He had hoped through this experimentation to develop an anti-Syphilis vaccine.[57] If it were not for Susan Reverby examining Cutler's private notes at the University of Pittsburgh in order to gain more insight into Tuskegee and its mechanics, the story of his involvement in and coordination of a Guatemalan experiment under the auspices of the US PHS and the Guatemalan Ministry of Health would not have come to light. Here 1500 prisoners, orphans and inmates of mental asylums were deliberately infected with Syphilis and gonorrhoea with up to one-third of them denied any treatment. Even though it shut down in 1948 (after only 2 years of field work), in some ways this study was even more shocking than Tuskegee because it sought to directly infect people who either didn't know what was happening or whose mental capacity wasn't sufficient to know.[58] Unlike the Sing Sing study, even though the Guatemalan work was so rakish that it was never published, it reminds one of the desire at the *fin-de-siècle* to '*Syphilize*' the French nation. What went on in Guatemala under the auspices of two governments would probably have made Joseph Auzias-Turenne quite proud indeed. These architects of Syphilis inoculation are thankfully now relegated to the academic dustbin of history.[59]

Sexually transmitted diseases (or at least their threat) would claim the job of the first African American Surgeon General, Joycelyn Elders in 1993 and '*Tuskegee by*

---

[57] The concept was that patients with prior exposure to Syphilis if injected with a high dose of spirochaetes and then observed would not become either reinfected or contagious.

[58] Reverby's work resulted in an official apology by then Secretary of State Hillary Clinton and the HHS secretary Kathleen Sibelius. In the study, direct inoculation of sexually transmitted diseases was made by skin contact, injection and abrasion of the face, arms, penis and cervix. Sexual congress between study subjects and known infected prostitutes was encouraged as prostitution (and their procurement for prisoners) was legal at the time in Guatemala. The co-coordinator on the Guatemalan end was PHS-trained Juan Funes, the Chief of the Guatemalan Sanidad Publica and graphic photos of the lesions induced were taken by Cutler's wife Eliese. The full story is even worse, where anti-convulsant (anti-epilepsy) therapy was traded for the right to inoculate some cases who were mentally retarded. [See SM Reverby. Ethical failure and History Lessons. The US Public Health Service Research Studies in Tuskegee and Guatemala. US PHS Inoculation Sexually Transmitted Disease (STD) Studies in Guatemala 1946–1948]. The data pertaining to the study is available online at the National Archives Records. A subsequent lawsuit was locally dismissed by virtue of Sovereign immunity but is currently being appealed. After these 'experiments' Cutler's career actually blossomed and he became Assistant Surgeon General in 1958.

[59] One other notable infamous example of coercive inoculation in American medical history includes the brainchild of Dr Chester Southam (1919–2002) an eminent immunologist at Sloan Memorial Hospital in New York. He injected cancer cells into elderly non-cancerous patients without their permission at the Jewish Chronic Diseases Hospital in Brooklyn in 1964 in order to further his research on immunological senescence and to define responses to cancer challenge in the elderly. This followed work he had already performed injecting a range of infective illnesses (including mumps, dengue fever, West Nile virus and Semliki Forest virus) into severely ill cancer patients. His cancer studies investigating the possibility that cancer was viral in origin started with the injection of leukemia victims (and also healthy Ohio State Penitentiary inmates) with purified cancer cells without informing them of the nature and content of the injections. Although Southam was officially sanctioned he ultimately became the President of the American Association of Cancer Research (1968–69).

association' (if you will) would claim her nominated replacement obstetrician Henry W. Foster Jr. In Elders' case, President Clinton fired her after her remarks that masturbation might be encouraged as an alternative to abstinence and in Foster's situation, it was presumed that as Vice President of the Macon County Medical Society (having attended CDC-related meetings), that he must have known of some details of the by then infamous Tuskegee study. Although the affidavits at the drawn out ending of the Tuskegee study on what Foster knew and when he knew it were conflicted, his nomination whilst making it through committee died in legislative limbo and his appointment was never voted upon.[60] The final impingement of Tuskegee on the executive branch of government would come with President Clinton's emotional White House apology on the 16th May 1996. The speech spawned a bioethics center, a museum of memory and the legislative will to include minorities in a national research agenda.[61]

Like all truths and reconciliations, Tuskegee has been distilled and reduced into something simpler and more blameworthy even if it appears less personalized than its Nuremberg predecessor. Its flawed ethos was itself a victim of the times that 'handled' African Americans within the Health Service and that reflected within the Justice system that differential response towards Blacks and Whites. Alongside Tuskegee, Americans witnessed the false imprisonment in 1931 of the Scottsboro boys over the alleged rape of two white women and the nation fitfully careened towards the Montgomery bus protest by Tuskegee's Rosa Parks when she refused in 1951 to surrender her seat. From then it lurched on to the assassinations of Martin Luther King and Malcolm X and thence to the Selma to Montgomery March that led to the Civil Rights Acts. Today the same racial issues and stereotypic responses have resurfaced following the street murder by the police of George Floyd and in the local backlash by Southern State legislatures confronting those who argue that the teaching of Critical Race Theory is an opportunity to open a national conversation about racial history in America. Even during those earlier changing times, intransigent PHS researchers like Joseph Earle Moore obsessed with his Syphilis projects in an era of effective treatment would callously lament that "*the biologically minded clinician regrets,* [however], *that syphilis seems to be vanishing with most of its fascinating and more fundamental riddles still unresolved*".[62]

---

[60] Foster's nomination was withdrawn after it became evident that he had performed many abortions and following a filibuster against the appointment run by the pro-life Republican Senator Phil Gramm.

[61] Concerning the Presidential apology, (although those whose original idea it was is debated), it was formally addressed on the floor of Congress immediately following Bill Clinton's 1996 re-election by the Congressional Black Caucus via Rep. Louis Stokes (1925–2015) of Ohio and Rep. Maxine Waters (1938-) of California. An apology from the State of Alabama to the Tuskegee families, however, was not forthcoming until 2001.

[62] Joseph Earle Moore. *Penicillin in Syphilis.* Springfield Ill. Charles C. Thomas. 1946: p. 147.

Chapter 7
Syphilocentricity in Brief: Disease in the Post-HIV Era

Abstract We have seen with COVID-19 a society dominated by the science of infection. In a sense in the face of a syphilitic landscape, the structure of that epidemic has been repeated. Similarly, the antimicrobial goal shifts from defeat of the organism to its attenuation and some form of cohabitation. A pandemic downgrades to an epidemic which then abates to an endemic manageable condition. With Syphilis, there is homology with the medical and social response to HIV-AIDS as well as to the war against COVID-19. Each has run through a comparable chronology of events that has included effective diagnostic testing, contact tracing and the development of a Zauberkügel. Syphilis has, however, been the least politicised of the 3 diseases and less derailed by those forces seeking to deny the role of science.

Looking back, any perception of success that we might have experienced against the *Treponeme* was always a reflection of our interpretation of its natural history. No triumph could have occurred isolated from the perspective that even with a magic bullet, its defeat (or more correctly its attenuation), could not have happened without consideration of the environment from which it sprang. Man as victim with all his social customs and his economy would always modify the disease itself.

In all the editorials of the *New York Times* throughout the eventful year of 1910 which highlighted Paul Ehrlich's great discovery Salvarsan, none had called Syphilis by its name. In Ehrlich's time, Syphilis affected between 5 and 10% of the adult population of Europe and was the cause of one-third of the cases of insanity confined to mental asylums. It was thought responsible for about a quarter of stillbirths and the same number of stunted feeble-minded infants. From the time of the Ancien régime, syphilitics (and their progeny) were an existential threat and for some tore at the very fabric that the tenets of the new philosophy had prescribed for any group which regarded itself as civilized.

The history of Syphilis is, however, more than its prevention, diagnosis and cure. To merely imagine Syphilis in this restrictive manner confines it like any other illness almost to the realm of an abstraction. Something totally defined by its biology and dominated by its laboratory characteristics, its clinical manifestations and the strategies for its defeat. This is the *Biological Syphilis* and is only one way of looking at it. But Syphilis has many guises. It is paradigmatic and all such illness lies in singular disequilibrium with its community. Its perceptions are societal perceptions and its history more an historiography.

However Syphilis orchestrated its arrival, it took on the character of an epidemic, although as a distinctly biological event it is unique with neither a readily recognizable beginning nor an apparent end. All it reasonably can be said to have possessed was an observable middle. Syphilis persists today without comprehensive defeat. The way we imagine our response to it, however, sits very differently to our retrospective impression of how we have managed viruses like poliomyelitis or smallpox.[1] In his 1962 book *The Cholera Years*, Charles Rosenberg examines cholera outbreaks in the United States in 1832, 1849 and 1886[2] and his proposed taxonomy of the different sorts of epidemics draws parallels with our historical understanding of Syphilis as a disease. At the commencement of any pestilential scourge the search for presumptive causes as an explanation for widespread suffering moved (for Rosenberg), from the first impression that it was an affliction sent by God to one which quickly laid blame upon some maligned minority group. The first fear is retributive and penitential, the second distinctly blameworthy and directed more frequently at a country's most recent immigrants or even at its own indigenous population. As societies might imagine themselves more evolved, the responsibilities and jurisdictions of the prefectures to provide clean water then caused a decline in the number of cases of a range of infective diseases like cholera, typhoid and Tuberculosis in the major towns and cities. These declines came well before each illness had either an attributable organism or a specific anti-bacterial magic bullet. These were what one might call epidemics of hygiene now characterized by a communitarian 'sanitational' reactivity. Finally, only afterwards would medical advances assuage the epidemic, identifying the culpable microorganism, establishing simple and widely reproducible tests for the diagnosis of prior or current exposure and ultimately discovering specific targeting antibiotics for clinical use. The medical response to such an epidemic threat was logistical.

If first the epidemic was the province and interest of a vengeful Deity, only then did it point an accusatory finger at society's most vulnerable and disenfranchised. Response would occur to a social crisis which was capable of being contained with regular metropolitan legislation and it would finally counter the alien antigen by unleashing the power of medical science. Once science could engage it was

---

[1] Some viruses have been eradicated by using stimulating vaccinial lookalikes either as the killed products of the virus or as attenuated whole viruses. This is not an option for Syphilis. Vaccination against Syphilis cannot currently be achieved as it has no animal reservoir and the organism cannot be propagated in the laboratory (what is called *in vitro*) for any sustainable length of time (although it has been carried into short-term cell culture). The coding of the genome of the *Treponema pallidum* raised some hopes of a genetically-modified vaccine but initial trialing of syphilitic proteins failed to provide immunity in animal studies.

[2] Charles Rosenberg. *The Cholera Years. The United States in 1832, 1849 and 1866*. University of Chicago Press. 1987.

expected that an experimental method would incrementally but ultimately catch up with the Syphilis microbe. This was anticipated even when on occasion science itself had sailed away from accepted ethical conventions. Therefore, once the bacillus was visualized under the microscope in 1905, some of its fate was already sealed. Only a wily bacterial mutational flexibility and its fastidious insistence on living freely amongst humans in the face of the destructive power of Penicillin has somehow saved it from complete annihilation. Unlike other bacteria, it could not evolve the machinery of antibiotic resistance but yet it presented if only by mollifying its power to kill to an affliction that today is more of an embarrassment than anything else. The move by the spirochaete from lethality to intrusiveness seems a heavy price to pay for its organic survival.

But we see that the history of Syphilis has been much more; even a concentrated polemic about lifestyle. The fight against it has been overly imbued with religious and political overtones which at times have overpowered an ability to treat it or to restrict its spread. Indeed frequently the concerted public health response against it has been a virtual referendum on sexuality itself. After bursting on to the world stage, HIV/AIDS too once it had been defined became a disease of the activists in a way Syphilis could never be and permitted a greater engagement by its victims in the trajectory of research and care and in the shaping of public health policy. Comparing the social and medical response to Syphilis, the focus in the case of HIV/AIDS moved from disease identification to disease attenuation with comparatively remarkable speed. Syphilis drew considerable ire as did the emergence of HIV/AIDS from a society intolerant of homosexuality even if with Syphilis there had been so little description of its spread throughout the 18th and 19th Centuries other than by hetrerosexual encounters.[3] Its risk was seemingly only tenuously linked to the romantic notions in the imagination of the poets of rhapsodized trysts between cultured mentors and impressionable boys and young men.

But both diseases retained their specialized status because of the sexualization of each although AIDS would always adopt a more human face.[4] Both would induce the best and the worst of community responses with AIDS sufferers receiving from one hand the help of community support groups and the benefits of an education

---

[3] William Benemann. *Male—Male Intimacy in Early America: Beyond Romantic Friendships.* Binghamton New York Haworth Press 2006; pp. 135–138 quoted in John Parascandola. Ch 6. *Magic in the Face of Penicillin: Syphilis in America since World War II.* pp. 132–154 In John Parascandola (Ed). *Sex, Sin and Science: A History of Syphilis in America.* Healing Society: Disease Medicine and History. Westport CT Praeger 2008].

[4] The NAMES Project Foundation quilt is a particular example supplementing new panels in homage to the victims of HIV-AIDS by region as they fell. It became the largest cooperative art project in the world.

drive but losing freedoms on the other through the quarantine of some cases and the basic threat that public exposure placed upon privacy.[5] Even those religious groups offering their assistance through hospices would be the most vociferous opponents of the distribution of condoms and would appear on occasion to abet the criminalization of each illness. Two centuries on, the punitive parallels with the Parisian Bicêtre hospital shackling its syphilitic women to their beds in its squalid wards, are stark indeed.

If Sir Jonathan Hutchinson had labeled Syphilis '*the great imitator*' then by this definition alone it might (albeit somewhat archaically) remain part of any modern differential diagnosis. But Syphilis is defined by context and even today is potentially capable of shifting its shape. With a rise in the number of new Syphilis cases amongst gay and bisexual men, Syphilis has today become a hydra exploiting other infectious agents through fortuitous sexual encounters as its latest and ablest springboard.[6] Today with Syphilis we see a repeat of the inverse paradox of yesteryear. In some undeveloped countries its prevalence rises whilst communication about its dangers can often be suppressed. Now it is only a shadow of an ancient terror, settling into a softer venereal disease after early on, killing too many of its hosts. Even the very nature of the bacillus is obscure. Is it one or a number of subtypes and why has it developed a link so close to humans, uniquely hitching its evolution to ours so that it cannot survive away from us for any length of time or in any preservative culture medium? The rash of complex and bizarre neurological cases of a specialized and grandiose dementia only appeared in the 19th Century and this too may have represented a specific mutation that created an entirely new component to an old malady. So too in its neurological destruction, the converse profusion of *fin-de-siècle* syphilitic geniuses may have been the hallmark of such a genetic change in the bacillus that only became apparent amongst the glut of stiflingly prudish Victorian and Edwardian literature.[7] Only the Romanian essayist Emil Cioran (1911–1995) would openly profess his '*Syphilis envy*' yearning for a

---

[5] A concept suggested by David L Kirp (University of California-Berkeley) and Ronald Bayer (Columbia University) *AIDS in the Industrialized Democracies: Passions, Policies.* New Brunswick NJ Rutgers University Press. 1992.

[6] Genital ulceration by Syphilis may promote the absorption and progression of the HIV virus.

[7] Another example is provided by Thomas Mann in *Dr. Faustus: The Life of the German Composer Adrian Leverkühn, Told by a Friend* (*Doktor Faustus: Das Leben des deutschen Tonsetzers Adrian Leverkühn, erzählt von einem Freunde*) written between 1943 and 1947 where a composer in a tryst with the Devil contracts Syphilis confined to his central nervous system. It provokes a portfolio of creative genius for the next 24 years.

contagious brush with death if only it would osmotically transfer to him its productive literary genius.[8]

Today, Syphilis is a quite uncommon cause of illness in developed countries and
with antibiotic attenuation its opportunity to invade the central nervous system has
been severely curtailed. Despite this, it rears its head now with a 50-fold increase in
its incidence in the Federated Soviet States. Indeed, its incidence appears to be
rising. With the freer movement from the Russian borders we have seen its convivial expansion into Northern Europe, the United States and Israel tracing the
movement of Soviet émigrés. The other way of looking at Syphilis is of course
conceptually. The idea of illness (in the absence of any known causation), was as
John Donne (1572–1631) had written in his 1627 *Devotions Upon Emergent
Occasions*,[9] one where survival would appear only as small cracks in a fortress
wall. Donne had written his poem when he thought that he was dying (possibly of
typhus or of relapsing fever although his precise illness is unknown). Each of his
structured stanzas played firstly with his devout meditations which led then to the
strongest sermonizing and ultimately to penitential prayer. For Donne, the battle
with disease was always the inexorable battle with sin. Identification of the
microscopic nature of disease changed all that, but the war against Syphilis would
always look metaphorically like any conflict, claiming its collateral victims many of
whom because of the sexualization of disease would not command any public
sympathy.

The medical historian Allan Brandt has suggested (as have many others) that
Syphilis and HIV/AIDS in their chronology and reactions share much in common.[10] Both have suffered from a panicked fear of contagion, the casual nature in
some cases of their transmission, a societal stigmatization following diagnosis and
the transgression of the civil liberties of their sufferers. In both cases, there was
perhaps an overly optimistic anticipation of disease elimination after the discovery
of each one's magic bullet. Both upon the cusp of medical victory would suffer at
the hands of some who would suggest that the attendant publicity surrounding each

---

[8] See Susan Sontag. *AIDS and its Metaphors*. Farrar, Strauss & Giroux. 1989 p. 23. Also Willis G.
Regier. *Cioran's insomnia*. MLN December 2004; 119 (5): pp. 994–1012 Comparative Literature
Issue Johns Hopkins University Press. Cioran attributed his insomnia (as did his mother) "*like
genius, talent and melancholy...to masturbation and syphilis*". [See E. Cioran *Oeuvres*, Paris
Gallimard 1995; p. 235]. Cioran regarded afflictions such as intractable insomnia to be 'gifts' to his
prolific literary output. The American essayist Adam Gopnik attested that Cioran had claimed not
to have slept for 50 years. [See Adam Gopnik. The Get-Ready Man. In the New Yorker June 19th
2000; pp. 172–180].

[9] More exactly *Devotions Upon Emergent Occasions; and severall steps in my Sickness*.

[10] Allan M. Brandt. *No Magic Bullet. A Social History of Venereal Disease in the United States
Since 1880*. Oxford University Press 1985.

disease would promote a promiscuity that could only exacerbate the very problem others were trying devotedly to overcome.[11] And in this, many would also identify both diseases by their very physical expressions.[12] Brandt's prescriptions for society (if lessons can be learned), seem as immutable as Koch's postulates governing the infectious nature of disease and would seem as apposite for HIV/AIDS in the last decade as they would have been for Syphilis in the 19th Century. A public health policy driven by fear is unlikely to have sustained success and the best intended education and the clearest exposition of the latest available science on the subject can often be somewhat doomed in controlling the spread of disease. We have witnessed such corollaries during the recent waves of the COVID pandemic. Eradication of the microbe might be a laudable but an impossible and simplistic aim in a world where genetic changes may occur upon environmental stresses at any moment to produce drug resistance or the emergence of a new more frightening variant to which there is little population immunity. The new history the spirochaete could at least in theory create for itself (and from there its future clinical trajectory), will still be the legacy of our past mistakes.

The *Transformative Syphilis* is one where only a hindsight observation (whether that be historical or genetic) can reveal its prior evolution. Both history and molecular biology can modify our understanding of Syphilis as it moves through distinctly mutational events. The language of disease too influences our perception. In some illnesses like cancer, we describe responsiveness to treatment as regression although it is an inept word since tumours do not revert under stress to earlier simpler forms. They are defeated by the new agents targeting proteins that have lost their defense to molecular destruction. So too do we describe the regression of Syphilis to a more manageable and less intrusive disease although we do not understand its defining mutational schisms. It is expected that future ecologies might compel the spirochaete to change again towards most likely some new aggression.

The body politic of Syphilis might also be considered to have some structure, possessing a head and a heart. At one time, the dimension of a *Political Syphilis* terrifyingly embraced a social Darwinism that had its treatment resources denied to ethnic groups thought either unworthy or inferior. Its false head became wrapped up in meetings that justified the denial of therapy in the Tuskegee experiment and

---

[11] For some groups, throughout history, it has been argued that those advocating safer sex practices are actually promoting promiscuity. [See Perry Treadwell. *Gods, Judgment, Syphilis and AIDS*. San José CA Writers Club Press 2001]. This echoed the vehement old idea of Jean Astruc that some treatments (even if effective) were liable to lead to risky sexual practice writing in his 1754 *Treatise of the Venereal Disease* that *"once the fear of infection by which men are restrained for intemperance is removed, then the Reins of Lust will be let loose"*. [2 vols London] Vol. 1; p. 283.

[12] For some, regardless of the medical advances, Syphilis and AIDS are still considered punishments whose origins lie either in promiscuity or perversity. For these religious exponents, part of their argument lies in the physical retributions of 'ancient Syphilis' characterized by its destructive deformations of the faces of both children and adults as a reminder of its price. Sontag particularly mentions *'the aristocracy of the face'* which Syphilis fails to spare. [See Sontag *AIDS and its Metaphors Ibid*: p. 39].

which infused assumptions about a racial stereotype into a scientific anthropology blindly convinced that Black races were less likely to respond to curative therapies. Those assumptions were embedded into the wrong decisions that still haunt public health policy making today. By the time Tuskegee's own data debunked the idea of the aberrant physiology of the Negro, its own researchers still steadfastly denied the participants worthwhile treatment and by then they had surrendered their heart. The disease had been selfishly tied to the impression of an entire race thought incapable of mounting any sustained response and for some the Negro was on the road to obliteration. Refusing treatment might shamefully in the minds of those advocates just have helped that inevitable process along.

In his book *Death in the Afternoon*, Ernest Hemingway calls Syphilis "*an industrial accident...it is a to-be-expected end, or rather phase, of the life of all fornicators.*" [13] It is a disease which through its own iconic power changed sexual experience from a licentious abandon to a moralizing oppression and then back again. HIV/AIDS is locked in a similar sexualizing transition. The place of Syphilis in current society lies (as Sontag suggests) in the predictive capacity of its future rather than with its past. [14] In times ahead, how such disease will seem depends upon how close to right our analyses have been today. Only hindsight of its completed evolution will either strengthen or dispel our current commentaries. It appears as we are conquering AIDS that like the triumph over Syphilis with its magic bullets, that the extraordinary nature of illness (and even its supernatural elements) have been tamed into something inherently prosaic. [15] The character of venereal disease will neither develop (nor regress) in a social vacuum. It will always be tethered to how we view sexual practices and to our embrace of sexual and gender diversity and identity. Syphilis with its capacity to 'pandemicize', today lies dormant. But it has always been an illness encoded by the tension between rational science and reacting religious and political belief systems. Whether it will once again mutate and dominate social discourse through its physical impact, remains to be seen. In such a freshly 'syphilocentric' world there will need to be a new polemic where future cultural messages will become the latest vector for a changed micro-organism. No doubt, in whatever form it takes, in the meantime Syphilis will continue to inspire in all the genres of the arts.

---

[13] Hemingway, Ernest. *Death in the Afternoon*. Charles Scribner & Sons 1932.

[14] Sontag. *Ibid* p 93. It is of value to re-examine her dissertation as HIV-AIDS has become more medicinally manageable where she correctly predicted the likelihood that it would 'de-dramatize' as a social illness.

[15] A similar transition is the ultimate challenge in how we will come to view cancers.

Bibliography

Armstrong J (1709–1779) Oeconomy of Love (1736). English Poetry. Fulltext dbase. Pt II. 1600–1800. Cambridge Engl: Alexandria Va. Chadwick-Healy;1994.

Astruc J. A treatise on the venereal diseases in six books containing an account of the origins, propagation and contagion of this distemper. Transl William Barrowby MD 1737. Reprint New York: Da Capo Press;1972.

Auzias-Turenne J-A. La syphilization. Paris: Études Poulain d/Andecy;1878.

Brandt AM. No magic bullet. A social history of venereal disease in the United States since 1880. Oxford University Press;1985.

Baudelaire C. Sur la Belgique, epilogue, complete works, vol. 2. le Dantec, Y-G. editors. Rev. by Claude Pichois: 1976.

Benemann W. Male-male intimacy in early America: beyond romantic friendships. Binghamton New York: Haworth Press;2006.

Bockenheimer P. Atlas der Chirurgischen Hautkrankheiten illustrating interesting surgical conditions. New York: Rebman;1913. A Collection of Coloured Plates.

Braslow J. Mental ills and bodily cures: psychiatric treatment in the first half of the 20th century. Berkeley University of California Press;1997.

Brasol B. Oscar Wilde: the man, the artist, the martyr. New York: Octagon;1975.

Bynum WF. Medical fringe and medical orthodoxy 1750–1850. Bynum WF, Porter R, editors. London: Croom Helm;1987.

Camus A. La Peste;1947.

Cellini B. The life of Benvenuto, son of master Giovanni Cellini, the Florentine. Written by himself in Florence, vol. 2, 1927 ed. The Navarre Society: London;1500–1571.

Cioran E. Oeuvres. Paris: Gallimard;1995.

Cowley RLS. Marriage à la mode: a review of Hogarth's Narrative Art. Manchester. Manchester University Press;1983.

Daudet A. In The Land of Pain (transl Julian Barnes). Knopf;2003, 1930.

Daudet L. Les Morticoles. 1894.

Daudet L. Devant la douleur. 1915 ed.

Debus AG. The chemical philosophy and alchemy book. New York: Science History Publications;1977.

Defoe D. Fortunes and misfortunes of the famous Moll Flanders. 1722. Ed Starr GA editor. London: Oxford University Press;1971.

De Maupassant G. Complete short stories of Guy de Maupassant. New York: Doubleday;1955.

Devergie M-N. Clinique de la maladie syphilitique. Enrichie d'observations communiqués par Messieurs Cullerier oncle, Cullerier neveu, Bard, Gama, Desruelles et autre mèdecins, vol. 2. Paris F-M Maurice;1826–1833 (Atlas).

Dinesen I, (Blixen K). The Third Cardinal's Tale. (In The Last Tales). New York: Vintage;1957.

Donaldson-Evans M. Medical examinations: dissecting the doctor in French narrative prose. 1857–1894. Lincoln University of Nebraska;2000.

Donne J. Devotions upon emergent occasions; and severall steps in my sickness.

Dulaure JA. Histoire de Paris. Guillaume Paris;1821–1825.

Eder FX. Sexual cultures in Europe: themes in sexuality. In: Eder FX, Hall LA, Hekma G, editors. Manchester and New York: Manchester University Press;1999.

Elder AL. The history of Penicillin production. New York: American Institute of Chemical Engineers;1970.

Fildes V. Wet-nursing: a history from antiquity to the present. Oxford Basil: Blackwell;1988.

Gjestland T. The Oslo study of untreated syphilis: an epidemiologic investigation of the natural course of the syphilitic infection based upon a re-study of the Boeck-Brussgaard material. Akademisk Forlag;1955.

Goldhagen DJ. Hitler's willing executioners. Ordinary Germans and the Holocaust. Vintage Books 1997. Hitlers willige Vollstrecker: Ganz gewöhnliche Deutsche und der Holocaust-German Edition.

Goldwater LJ. Mercury: a history of quicksilver. Baltimore: York Press;1972.

Grob GN. The mad among us: a history of the care of America's mentally ill. New York: Free Press;1994.

Guillemeau J. The manual of nursing and bringing up of children. 1612 Reprint New York: Da Capo Press;1972 Ed.

Hayden D. Pox: genius, madness and the mysteries of syphilis. Basic Books;2003.

Harlan L. The secret life of Booker T. Washington. In: Raymond WS, editor. Washington in perspective, essays of Louis R Harlan. Jackson University Press of Mississippi;1988.

Hemingway E. Death in the afternoon. Charles Scribner and Sons;1932.

Hobby G. Penicillin. Meeting the challenge. New Haven CT: Yale University Press;1985.

Hutchinson J. Syphilis. London, Paris, New York: Cassell and Co;1887.

Jones JH. Bad blood. The Tuskegee syphilis experiment. Free Press;1982.

Kipling R. The many inventions. 1893.

Kirp DL. (University of California-Berkeley) and Ronald Bayer (Columbia University) AIDS in the industrialized democracies: passions, policies. New Brunswick NJ: Rutgers University Press;1992.

Klotz O. Diary notes on a trip to West Africa in relation to a Yellow Fever expedition under the auspices of the Rockefeller Foundation of 1926. Brentano's;1926.

Lagerkvist Ulf. Pioneers of microbiology and the Nobel Prize. New Jersey: World Scientific;2003.

Lederer S. Subjected to science. Human experimentation in America before the Second World War. Johns Hopkins University Press;1995.

Leoniceno N. De Morbo Gallico. Milan Venice;1497.

Lewis JH. The biology of the Negro. Chicago: Chicago University Press;1942.

McBride D. From TB to AIDS: Epidemics among urban Blacks since 1900. Albany: SUNY Press;1991.

McGough LJ. Gender, sexuality and syphilis in early modern Venice. The disease that came to stay. Rab Houst, Edward Muir: Palgrave MacMillan;2010.

Margulis L. Symbiotic planet: a new look at evolution. Basic Books;1998.

Marks HM. The progress of experiment: science and therapeutic reform in the United States 1900–1990. Cambridge Studies in the History of Medicine;2001.

Marquhardt M. Paul Ehrlich. Introduction by Sir Henry Dale: William Heinemann Medical Books Ltd.; 1949.

May HF. The end of American innocence: a study of the first years of our own time. New York: Columbia University Press;1912–1917.

Merians LE. The secret malady. Venereal disease in eighteenth Century Britain and France. Merians LE, editor. University Press of Kentucky;1996.

Montesquieu, L'esprit des lois 1748.

Moore JE. Penicillin in syphilis. Springfield Ill. Charles C. Thomas;1946. The modern treatment of syphilis, 2nd ed. Springfield Ill. Charles C. Thomas: 1947.

Mracek F. Atlas of syphilis and the venereal diseases, including a brief treatise on the pathology and treatment. Lemuel Bolton Bangs. Philadelphia WB Saunders;1898.

Nabarro DN. Congenital syphilis. London E. Arnold;1934.

Oppe AP. Thomas Rowlandson: his drawings and watercolours. London: The Studio Ltd;1923.

Parascandola, J. Sex sin and science. A history of syphilis in America. Praeger Westport;2008.

Perrett DB. Ethics and error: the dispute between Ricord and Auzias-Turenne over syphilisation 1847–1870. Thesis Stanford University;1977.

Quétel, C. History of syphilis. Johns Hopkins University Press Baltimore;1990.

Ransome A. Oscar Wilde: a critical study. Mitchell Kennerley New York: Dedicated to Robert Ross;1912.

Reverby SM. Tuskegee truths: rethinking the Tuskegee Syphilis Study. University of North Carolina Press;2000. Examining Tuskegee. The infamous syphilis study and its legacy. The John Hope Franklin Series in African American History and Culture. University of North Carolina Press;2009.

Ricord P. Lettres sur la syphilis. Paris L'Union Médicale;1865.

Rosahn PD. Autopsy studies in syphilis. Washington D.C. PHS 1949 Publication.

Rosenberg C. The Cholera years. The United States in 1832, 1849 and 1866. University of Chicago Press;1987.

Russell B. The History of Western Philosophy. London: Unwin Publishers;1979 (1946 1st ed.).

Schamberg JF, Wright CS. Treatment of syphilis. New York Appleton;1932.

Sherard, R. Oscar wilde: the story of an unhappy friendship. London: Hermes Press;1902.

Sheridan RH. The life, work and evil fate of Guy de Maupassant. New York Brentano's:1926.

Smith WG. The amorous illustrations of Thomas Rowlandson. London Bibliophile Books;1983.

Shweder R. The idea of moral progress. Bush vs Posner vs Berlin. Philosophy of Education Year Book. Urbana Ill. Philosophy of Education Society.

Sontag S. Illness as Metaphor. 1978. Farrar, Strauss and Giroux New York AIDS and its Metaphors: Farrar, Strauss and Giroux;1989.

Spitz V. Doctors from Hell. Sentient Publications;2005.

Steegmuller F. The letters of Gustave Flaubert (1830–1857). G. Flaubert and Francis Steegmuller: Bellknap Press; 1980.

Stone L. Family sex and marriage in England 1500–1800. New York: Harper and Row;1972.

Strahan SAK. Marriage and disease: a study of heredity and the more important family degenerations. London: Kegan Paul, Trench, Tribner & Co;1892.

Sudhoff K. The earliest printed literature on Syphilis. Being Ten Tractates from the years 1495–1498. Adapted by C. Singer Lier Florence. 1925.

Sussman G. Selling mother's milk: the wet-nursing business in France. 1715–1914. Urbana University of Illinois Press;1982.

Swift J. Gulliver's Travels. 1726 a.k.a. Travels into Several Remote Nations of the World. In Four Parts. By Lemuel Gulliver, First a Surgeon, and then a Captain of Several Ships, 2nd ed. Paul Turner Oxford: Oxford University Press;1986.

Thurston H. Butler's lives of the Saints. Thurston H, Attwater D, editors. vol. 4, 2nd ed. London: Burnes and Oates.

Treadwell P. Gods, judgment, syphilis and AIDS. San José CA: Writers Club Press;2001.

Vasari G. Lives of the Most Excellent Painters, Sculptors and Architects 1550.

Versluis A. The secret history of Western sexual mysticism: sacred practices and spiritual marriage. Destiny Books;2008.

Voltaire. L'homme aux quarante écus 1768. Candide 1759.

von Hutten U. De guiaci medicina et morbo gallico. Mainz 1519. Of the wood called guiacaum. London: Thomas Bertehelentregii;1540.

Werner Laurie T. The life of Oscar Wilde. 1906.

Werner Laurie T. The real Oscar Wilde. 1917.

Weindling PJ. Nazi medicine and the Nuremberg trials: from medical war crimes to informed consent. Palgrave Macmillan;2005.

Williams RC. United States Public Health Service 1798–1950. Published 1951.